A Catechism for Health Care

A Catechism
for Health Care

INSIGHTS FROM CATHOLIC TEACHING ON

Human Life, Medical Ethics, *and* Love of Neighbor

Edited by **STEPHEN NAPIER**
and **JOHN M. TRAVALINE**

The Catholic University of America Press
Washington, D.C.

Nihil Obstat:
Reverend J. Daniel Mindling OFM Cap., S.T.D.
Censor Deputatus

Imprimatur:
Most Reverend Juan Esposito, J.C.D.
Vicar General and Moderator of the Curia

The Roman Catholic Archdiocese of Washington
May 17, 2024

The *nihil obstat* and *imprimatur* are official declarations that a book or pamphlet
is free of doctrinal or moral error. There is no implication that those who have
granted the *nihil obstat* and the *imprimatur* agree with the content, opinions or
statements expressed therein.

The paper used in this publication meets the minimum requirements of American
National Standards for Information Science—Permanence of Paper for Printed
Library Materials, ANSI Z39.48-1992.

Cataloging-in-Publication Data is available from the Library of Congress
ISBN (paperback): 978-0-8132-3834-0
ISBN (ebook): 978-0-8132-3835-7

Book design by Burt&Burt
Text typeset in Minion Pro and Astoria

Dedication

SN:
To Carol and Katherine

JMT:
To Giovanni, Lucia, and Filomena,
having so much still to learn

Acknowledgments

Part of this project was made possible by the Veritas Award provided by the Office of the Provost at Villanova University. Stephen Napier and John Travaline would like to thank everyone at the Catholic University of America Press for helping us bring this work to fruition. We especially thank John B. Martino for shepherding this project to completion and especially for his contributions to the introduction. We thank Louise A. Mitchell for her insightful additions and corrections throughout the entire work. And we thank Brian Roach who has crafted a beautiful presentation to match the content of the book.

Contents

3. Genetics

4. The Body and Bodily Dimension of Sexual Love

5. Vaccines and Vaccination

6. At the End of Life

A Plea for Love

Moral Obligations and Options

Organ Donation

9. Conflicts of Interest

10. On the Role of Physicians, and the Patient–Physician Relationship

Introduction

The Church's Role in Health Care

"When John the Baptist heard in prison what the Christ was doing, he sent word by his disciples and said to him, 'Are you the one who is to come or are we to wait for another?' Jesus answered them, 'Go and tell John what you hear and see: the blind receive their sight, the lame walk, the lepers are cleansed, the deaf hear, the dead are raised, and the poor have great news brought to them'" (Mt 11:2–5 NRSV). The argument that Jesus uses to demonstrate that he is the Christ—the Anointed One promised to save Israel—is that he cared for the sick. Jesus knew what argument would be most persuasive to John the Baptist and should be most persuasive to us. Caring for the sick is deeply ensconced in being Christlike.

Healthcare delivery is an essential feature of the Church's mission, and the work of that mission is loving the sick and vulnerable. The first sentence of the *New Charter for Health Care Workers* reads, "The activity of healthcare workers is basically a service to life and health, which are primary goods of the human person. To this service is dedicated the professional or volunteer activity of those who are involved in various ways in preventive medicine, treatment, and rehabilitation."[1] Healthcare delivery is a direct service to the good of the human person.

Many, if not all, Catholic healthcare institutions employ not only ethicists, but also mission officers whose duties are to ensure that their

---

1 Pontifical Council for Pastoral Assistance to Health Care Workers, *New Charter for Health Care Workers*, trans. National Catholic Bioethics Center (Philadelphia: National Catholic Bioethics Center, 2017), 1.

hospital loves the sick and vulnerable as best they can. This includes, of course, loving those who work for such institutions and who execute her mission, and it also includes loving the surrounding community. According to the Internal Revenue Service, there are eight categories of community benefit. According to the Catholic Health Association, Catholic healthcare delivery accounts for the following:[2]

- $2.8 billion in financial assistance at cost (1), or charity care (2)
- 6.51 billion for unreimbursed Medicaid and other means test programs (3)
- $1.87 billion for community health improvement (4), subsidized health services (5), and in-kind contributions for community benefit (6)
- $1.8 billion for health professions' education (7)
- $547 million for healthcare-related research (8)

As impressive as these numbers are, the essence of Catholic health care is that the individual person is never reduced to a number. The dignity of every human person is the foundational reality for all of the Church's healthcare activity. Returning to the Gospel, Matthew records these words of Jesus, "for I was hungry and you gave me food, I was thirsty and you gave me something to drink, I was a stranger and you welcomed me, I was naked and you gave me clothing, I was sick and you took care of me, I was in prison and you visited me" (Mt. 25:35–36 NRSV). Our service to the hungry, the thirsty, the stranger, the naked, and the sick "is not only service to Christ himself, but representative of the kind of life that separates the sheep from the goats—from those who will have union with God forever and ever and those who will not."[3]

We begin with these reflections on Scripture to underscore the central concern of Catholic healthcare delivery, even though the complexities of delivering care in contemporary society can easily allow this biblical foundation to become obscured. Clinicians are asked to provide therapies for their patients, but as researchers, their goal is to get valid scientific knowledge; some clinicians may have interests as shareholders in a pharmaceutical company or device manufacturer, and still further,

2 Catholic Health Association, "Catholic Health Care: Community Benefit," April 2023, https://www.chausa.org/docs/default-source/community-benefit/cha-community-benefit-fact-sheet-2023.pdf.

3 Alisha N. Mack and Charles C. Camosy, *Bioethics for Nurses: A Christian Moral Vision* (Grand Rapids, Mich.: Wm. B. Eerdmans Publishing, 2022), 55.

clinicians in some areas have discipline-specific ethics codes that deviate from what would truly respect the human person. These diverse roles and competing expectations pull the clinician in different directions, setting up numerous points at which ethical conflict and moral distress could occur.

These same conflicts of interest can occur at the institutional level as well. For example, a hospital may have conflicting interests with the larger healthcare system of which it is a part because the hospital is in an area in which indigent care is a notable portion of its patient population. Other examples include Catholic–secular healthcare institutions in a joint venture or relationships with insurance companies such as Medicare. Sailing the seas of contemporary healthcare delivery can be rough with frequent crosswinds. Keeping on course requires attention and having a firm understanding of one's personal and institutional moral goals. The goal of this book is to help both institutions and individuals follow sound navigational guidance; namely, the principles offered by the teaching of the Catholic Church that help tune our own moral compasses to the true and good way to act in any circumstance.

Underlying many of the apparent dilemmas in health care is the question of what our goal really is. It is agreed by all that a healthcare institution needs to make money to stay in operation, but the motive for profit can nevertheless compromise patient care. The ethical dilemma here is not, however, between money and patient well-being. The reason is that profit contributes to staying in operation *so that* patients can be cared for. Moneymaking is not inconsistent with patient well-being. The ethical problem is not "balancing" these two goods, but discerning how best to ensure patient well-being with an eye towards charitable stewardship. As Jesus says in Matthew 6:24, we cannot serve two masters. Either we love God and hence our patients, and make use of money to provide them with care, or else we love "mammon" and hence our money, and make use of our patients to gain wealth.

In what follows, we explain the core themes in Catholic moral reflection the goal of which is to paint a picture of a moral vision that Catholic healthcare institutions and their clinicians can aspire to realize. Our hope is that you will think of the Church's moral guidance as not a list of "don'ts," or even a list of shoulds, but an encouragement towards a *beautiful* life amidst the inevitable pains and trials of the world. While there are clear "don'ts" and there are definitely "shoulds," we want to underline in this opening section that the whole picture of loving one's neighbor by providing health care is something that inspires us, and we hope will inspire you.

Core Themes in Catholic Moral Teaching

Deep in the caverns of the writings of the great medieval writer Thomas Aquinas is the following observation: "For we do not offend God except by doing something contrary *to our own good*."[4] Saint Thomas is quite clear that when we sin, we have done something contrary to our own benefit. Conversely, a virtuous life is the truly flourishing life, the happy life, the life that can act well with ease and contentment even in the midst of life's inevitable burdens. As far as Christian morality is concerned, the dividing line between vice and virtue is this: which course of action redounds to the benefit of the human person? By contrast, the popular stereotype of Christian morality can be seen if one were to cross out the phrase "our own good" and fill in the blank with something that sounds stricter. Many people might complete that sentence by inserting something like "God's law," "irrational rules," or "things to make me feel guilty."[5] Many view the Church's teachings, in fact, as positing that *only* actions that go *contrary* to our desires can actually be good. We typically think that we have to choose between morality and our desires—and if past generations chose duty, our generation chooses desire, the satisfaction of which we believe leads to happiness.

In truth, though, the Church's view of morality is that our own flourishing is at stake, as well as that of those we assist. If we have to say no to some of our desires, at least some of the time, that is because our immediate desires might not be properly informed or regulated by reason. The things we want to do today may not conform to what we deeply and truly long for—it is much more enjoyable to be healthy, for instance, but we might be tempted to eat today in a way that leads us to poor health. We all experience that, as intelligent animals in a complicated world, we may want many different things that we can't have all at once, or even that completely conflict with one another. Somehow we have to sort out which desires are helpful towards our flourishing and which desires are going to undermine it. To make those judgments, we often look to our families, to our friends, and to the messages of our

---

4 St. Thomas Aquinas, *Summa contra gentiles*, bk. 3, *Providence: Part II*, trans. Vernon J. Bourke (Notre Dame, Ind.: University of Notre Dame, 1975), 122.2 (emphasis added).

5 We owe these points to John M. Haas.

broader culture. But it just so happens that our contemporary culture is built around trying to sell us things—sometimes very good things, but often things that are not important or even are quite bad for us. Within a culture built around buying and selling almost everything—including human bodies—where do we find a guide who can lead us out of the confusion and into the clarity that will put our desires in an order that allows us to live a meaningful and happy life?

This is how we should understand the Church's moral teachings—not as a set of laws preventing us from being free, but as a description of how the world really works, once we take into account the whole picture. That whole picture includes God, the value of every human person, the long-term perspective on happiness, and the importance of justice and community to each person's flourishing. How can we get a sense of that whole picture? Imagine the Catholic Church's moral teachings in analogy with a galaxy. Every galaxy rotates around an unimaginably large center whose pull holds it all together. The gravitational center of the Church's teaching is *love for the human person*. Whatever we are talking about, whether it is the just distribution of goods in a society, marriage and family life, the decisions at the end of life, or even the most controversial issues that touch health care—such as reproductive technologies, contraception, or abortion—we are ultimately discerning what loving the human person looks like in purest form.

When we look *along* the Church's teachings and not merely *at* them, we can peer back to a specific teaching's roots. For instance, if you know about the papal teaching letter *Humanae vitae*, you might know that it discusses and reiterates the Church's perennial teaching on contraception. But unless you actually read the letter, you might not know that it orients us to see the issue through the lens of "responsible parenthood." It is as if the Church is describing the core of what truly loving your children looks like, namely, to have an attitude of openness to their existence. Merely looking *at* the teaching delivers the judgment, "don't use artificial contraception."[6] Looking *along* the teaching is to see

---

6 The legal scholar John Noonan for instance, understands the question on contraception as follows, "On what terms may the generation of human life be controlled? ... Under what conditions may human beings have sexual intercourse?" Noonan, *Contraception: A History of Its Treatment by the Catholic Theologians and Canonists* (New York: New American Library, 1967), xiii. Though Noonan's work is incredibly informative on the history of this topic from an academic standpoint, these starting questions do not invite one to look along this teaching and to see how love for human

the generosity of welcoming children into a loving relationship, and the challenge and opportunity of approaching family planning in another way (namely, what is known as fertility awareness or natural family planning). While this is a very challenging teaching to many today, especially in the medical profession, it is interesting to see that Pope Paul VI, in writing *Humanae vitae*, accurately predicted many failures to love that afflict modern culture—such as marital infidelity, a lowering of respect for women by men, and the use of these means by governments to coerce their populations on matters of childrearing. He foresaw these troubles because the Church's vision for life and love suggested that this seemingly benevolent technology—artificial contraception—would break apart things (sex and childrearing) that flourish best together.[7]

The present collection partly aims to function as a reminder to bring the many complex and ethically fraught dimensions of health care back to this gravitational center. It is meant to serve as a "recollection," if you will, which is a term used to describe a common spiritual discipline. This *Catechism for Health Care* is not an official document of the Church— but it collates the Church's teachings from official documents on issues arising in healthcare delivery and biomedical research, so that their roots in the love for human persons can be manifest. The reader is invited to look along each quotation to its axiological center.

We hope that this emphasis on love as a guiding principle for health care will be appealing to many people, but we recognize that they may not be ready to accept all of the insights and particular answers offered by the teaching of the Catholic Church. Even if everyone agrees that it is good to love human persons, disagreement arises concerning what precisely one means by love. What values or goods does the term "love" refer to? What "counts" as loving a human person? Though these are big questions, the complete answers to which require extended philosophical reflection, we will offer the following observations.

On the Christian view of human excellence, the best things for us are those goods that fulfill our nature, the deepest dimensions of ourselves that underlie our truest longings. The highest part of our nature, as even

---

persons informs the Church's teaching. The focus is on the sexual act itself. This is understandable, there is nothing wrong with looking intently at the branches; it is a welcome reminder, however, to notice the roots from which they came.

7 For details on how these predictions can be shown to have come true, see JoAnn Alicia Foley Markette, "Considering Conversion: The Aftermath of Oral Contraceptives," *Linacre Quarterly* 85, no. 4 (2018): 331–38.

the ancient Greeks held, includes the capacity to reason; hence acting in accordance with right reason is good. While the care of the body is essential to the practice of health care, we believe that the best medical professionals also recognize that human beings have a deeper self—what many traditions call the soul—and these souls are fulfilled primarily by truth and love. The philosopher Eleonore Stump observes, "Aquinas shares with other thinkers in the Christian tradition that personal relationship is the genus within which the greatest goods for human beings fall."[8] Health care that cares for the whole person acknowledges this primacy of relationships for their patients' well-being, and it sees the doctor–patient relationship as a particular kind of caring human relationship, not merely a business or technical transaction.

Furthermore, the highest good for human persons is the relationship with the ultimate source of life, which is to say, union with God. That is what we are made for, and that is what truly fulfills us. Stump observes, "On Aquinas's views, the worst thing that can happen to a person is to become alienated from God."[9] It follows that the best thing that anyone—including any healthcare provider—can do is to help another reconcile with God. If this idea seems foreign to us as doctors, nurses, healthcare workers today, perhaps we need to re-evaluate how we think of our calling as healers in the tradition of Christ. Of course, it cannot be done without respecting the consciences of our patients of whatever faith tradition or none. Nor should it replace the sound care of the physical body which is the special expertise of healthcare professionals. Rather, it means recognizing the limits of the help that care for the body can provide, and openness for the patient to seek healing for the soul.

The time that we have a patient in our office or our hospital can be shorter or longer, but it is always temporary. But although death is ultimately certain for all of us, the Church proclaims the Good News that our existence is not temporary. And goods that extend to eternity are more fulfilling than goods that are experienced only temporarily. C.S. Lewis tells us that,

> Christianity asserts that every individual human being is going to live forever, and this must be either true or false. Now there are a good

---

8 Eleonore Stump, "Providence and the Problem of Evil." In *The Oxford Handbook of Aquinas*, ed. Brian Davies (New York: Oxford University Press, 2012), 403.

9 Ibid., 402.

many things which would not be worth bothering about if I were going to live only seventy years, but which I had better bother about very seriously if I am going to live forever.[10]

Goods that fulfill our nature as beings made in the image of God and destined for union with God, are those goods that should serve as the central focus of one's love for another. Love tries to bequeath to the beloved the highest goods.

Happiness, on the Christian view, is not the fulfillment of as many as possible of our distinct desires, especially bodily ones; such satisfaction may help or hinder our fulfillment but is certainly not identical with it. I might experience a desire to smoke a cigarette, or drink one scotch too many, or stay in a romantic relationship that is objectively demeaning. The fact that I desire such things does not mean either that they are morally permissible to pursue or that they will fulfill me. Indeed, we can be mistaken about the genuine features of our true fulfillment, mistaking momentary pleasure or short-term comfort for genuine peace. Again, St. Thomas Aquinas is a helpful guide on these matters.

> Happiness is the final perfection of a human being. But everything is perfect to the extent to which it is in actuality, for potentiality is imperfect without actuality. Consequently, happiness must consist in the final actuality of a human being.[11]

The term "actuality" here refers to the exercise or operation of those capacities that are distinctive of the human person. Another way this is sometimes put is being "fully alive," or "living one's best life." These phrases, though, can lead us to imagine sitting on a beach in the Bahamas, sipping cocktails. This idea of the "good life"—as promoted by Caribbean cruise advertisements—could hardly explain why so many healthcare workers put on hospital gowns each day and wade into the fray of caring for patients. If this is why someone has joined the medical profession—to make millions and retire to a life of ease—it is highly likely that they won't last long enough in today's high stress environment to earn the money necessary for such a vision. Hence, it is probably true that, if you are working in health care, you have some idea of a higher

---

10 C.S. Lewis, *Mere Christianity* (New York: Touchstone Publishers, 1996), 73.

11 Thomas Aquinas, *Summa theologiae*, I, q. 3, a. 2, quoted in Eleonore Stump, *Aquinas: Arguments of the Philosophers* (New York: Routledge Publishers, 2004) 67.

notion of human fulfillment as well. We serve our neighbors because one of the highest capacities we have as human beings is entering into altruistic relationships, even with whatever stranger might appear at our door.

The Good News of Catholic health care is that the end of all of this service is not inevitably burnout or resentment, as so often seems the case today. If we serve as God intends, in truth and love, our service paradoxically can make us free—"whoever loses his life for my sake will find it," Jesus tells us (Mt 16:25). Indeed, it can enable us to know God as well as anyone can in this life. John the Evangelist says, "No one has ever seen God. Yet if we love one another, God remains in us, and his love is brought to perfection in us" (1 Jn 4:12). True fulfillment, then, should not be understood as some extravagant, inner religious experience, but the mundane working out of our love for others in concentric circles of influence: i.e., family, friends, local community, country, and so on. Happiness is realized in relationship, and the higher the being to which one is united, the greater the happiness. The unity here is best characterized as a symmetry of wills; when we will the same things God wills, we are oriented around the same goods that God "wants" realized. On this point, Stump observes (following Aquinas),

> You cannot get personal relationship with another person just by being in the same place as that person. You need also to have some meeting of minds and hearts, and there cannot be any such harmony of wills between a perfectly good God and a person whose will is not fixed in righteousness. It is in this way that there is distance between a human person and God.[12]

If disunity is a function of willing other than what God wills, unity is the converse; it is to have a symmetry of wills between oneself and God. One might say that what a good self-help book is for marriage, the Church's moral teachings are to one's union with God. The guidance is there, and if acted upon, leads to a greater union and relational happiness.

The guidance shared in this book is the teaching of the Church as best the editors could compile it, which will not answer every specific question in every moment of caring for the sick and injured. Nevertheless, it will exclude many false starts and wrong paths that are becoming

---

12 Eleonore Stump (with Jeffrey Tucker), "Beauty as a Road to God," *Sacred Music* 134, no. 4 (2007): 16.

all too common in a healthcare context built on bureaucracy, love of money, and concepts of the human person at odds with the one revealed in Scripture. By contrast to these opposing forces, Aquinas refers to love as willing the good of another. What is good for a human person? Whatever contributes to the person's flourishing. Flourishing means, among other things, the operation of one's distinctive capacities ordered to their proper ends. Loving another person involves willing that the beloved obtain the highest goods, and it also never violates their integrity.

It might help to see these concepts in action, as it were, on a specific and controversial issue. The Congregation for the Doctrine of the Faith promulgated an instruction titled *Persona humana* in which is addressed questions on sexuality. They state, "These final words briefly sum up the council's [Vatican Council II] teaching . . . on the finality of the sexual act and on the principal criterion of its morality: it is respect for its finality that ensures the moral goodness of this act."[13] The term "finality" is a precise philosophical expression that both medical professionals and the public may need explained. It does not mean the last part of an act, after which it is over. Rather, it means the ultimate purpose or meaning of something, its *raison d'etre* (reason for being), one may say. In the case of sexuality, even a rudimentary understanding of animal biology allows us to say that sexuality exists for the reproduction of the species. But the Church does not reduce human sexuality to the merely biological—we are, after all, animals with immortal, immaterial souls. Hence, the "finality" to which the council is referring, in the human case, is the potency of the sexual act to create another human being, another person who will live forever and its potency to bind the couple together through an act of mutual self-giving.

Respecting this "finality" means respecting the creative function of sex. Marriage is the context within which the good of the child can best be ensured, because of the educational and formative role that parents have in raising healthy children, who have the destiny of becoming good citizens on earth and children of God forever. It is reasonable, then, to order one's sexual choices in a way that respects the goods to which the sexual act is ordered, which is the rearing and caring for new human life and the unity of the spouses. Of course, not every sexual act must create a new life in order to be good; but the council's position is clear that the sexual act's *disposition* to create new human life must be respected in how

13 Congregation for the Doctrine of the Faith, *Persona humana*, V.

10

the act is carried out. It calls us to a high degree of sexual responsibility, so that we resist our immediate desires and any cultural encouragement to have intercourse in a context that cannot ensure a welcome home for new life. The point of the teaching is not merely to say, "do not have sex out of wedlock" (although it does say this). It is to direct one's mind to apprehend the beauty of a life that respects the goods inherent in one's actions, especially regarding something so precious and mysterious as the creation and education of new persons.

Though brief, these remarks describe the Church's basic moral conviction which is to see to it that human beings live flourishing lives. If a few pages of a book can do so, the editors hope this dispels the typical myths and stereotypes of the Church's teachings as merely constituting a list of "don'ts" forbidden by a legalistic God, or that the longing for happiness is foreign to the discipline of obeying the Church's teachings. At the root of the Church's teachings is a profound call to action namely, to will in oneself and in one's neighbor the greatest goods. Though the Church's teachings can be challenging to follow in certain circumstances, especially without the support of the prevailing culture, they are nevertheless the ingredients of a beautiful life. In fact, it is the Church's teaching that her moral teachings cannot be fully realized without God's grace, and that we are all very likely to fail and need forgiveness of sins on a regular basis. A spirit of acceptance when we fall short is what deprives pride of its lethal effects. When the editors ask students "what makes your best friends the best," they usually answer that the best are those who accept me, they are the person I can trust, and so on. The ability to forgive hurts is a huge part of that. The love for all human persons is reflexive; it means being a best friend to oneself, especially in view of moral setbacks.

In concluding this section on the Catholic moral vision, it is important to emphasize the Church's teaching on forgiveness and its corollary, acceptance of grief. This is mentioned here because of the secret suffering effected by, for example, post-abortion grief, and other psychological sequelae of not living up to one's moral ideals.[14] The best articulation of the Church's teaching on forgiveness is by a connoisseur of one who has experienced it. A participant named Molly at a Rachel's Vineyard

---

14 Grief is an emotion the follows a sense of loss. What is lost when we do not live up to our moral ideals is a sense of moral security and self-worth. As the text describes, restoring self-charity is an important effect of the forgiveness process.

retreat (a ministry for post-abortion mothers and fathers) describes her journey as follows:

> In a simple homily message, thirty plus years of denial about my abortion was awakened. I wondered, how did this priest know to reach into my heart and squeeze it? "God's desire," he said, "is to grant us mercy, forgiveness, and love, softening our hardened hearts so that we can repent and have eternal life with Him."[15]

Here we see two facts: The reason for the Church's teaching on abortion and other issues is because God loves us; the reason for the Church's teaching on forgiveness and the importance of *self*-charity is because God loves us. Saying that God is okay with killing vulnerable, nascent life is not to describe a loving God; saying that God does not desire to heal and unite with those who perform (or ask another to perform) such actions does not describe a loving God either. With an initial assurance that God desires union *with her*, Molly continues to describe her forgiveness process as follows:

> When I finally emptied myself of all the pain, I felt Jesus wrap his arms around me and weep with me. He took my hand and told me that He loved me and that I was forgiven. He asked me to forgive myself and told me that a very dear child in heaven was praying for me and was waiting to be reunited with me. When my tears and sobs slowed down, I found that all I hated in myself seemed to be dying, and thoughts of new life, filled with His love, rose up in me. He turned something ugly and sinful into a joyful and beautiful awakening of His love and mercy.[16]

The Church's Authority in Health Care

It was said of Jesus, "the crowds were astounded at his teaching, for he taught them as one having authority" (Mt 7:28b–29a). The Catholic Church, in continuity with her Master, teaches with authority through the office known as the Magisterium (which comes from the Latin

---

15 "Postabortion Healing: Letter from a Past Rachel's Vineyard Retreatant," *Life in Focus* newsletter (Fall 2009), https://www.rachelsvineyard.org/PDF/Articles/Post%20 Abortion%20Healing%20-%20Letter%20from%20Molly.pdf.

16 "Postabortion Healing: Letter from a Past Rachel's Vineyard Retreatant," *Life in Focus* newsletter (Fall 2009), https://www.rachelsvineyard.org/PDF/Articles/Post%20 Abortion%20Healing%20-%20Letter%20from%20Molly.pdf.

magister, meaning teacher). This authority is often unwelcome today, especially in light of the human failings of the Church's ministers in the realm of sexual abuse. It could be asked, "Why even bother with the Church's teaching?" in these enlightened, progressive times. While a full answer is impossible in a short introduction, we will offer a few possible responses.

To even the most skeptical reader, it should be said that the Magisterium of the Catholic Church has an impact on the world. It guides Catholic hospitals and other healthcare initiatives, not only in the United States but also around the world. Furthermore it guides the lives of many Catholic believers, who would rather suffer great penalties than to break God's commandments. The clear presentation of these teachings in this book should facilitate the understanding of this influential point of view.

The second point to note is that everyone has an authority. If one disagrees with the Church, one must trust one's own moral sensitivities more so than those who constitute the teaching function of the Church. Whether you agree or disagree, the ascription of an authority cannot be avoided. We can just as well ask, "Why should I listen to my own conscience? Why do I think that it is more reliable than others?" The point is more of a reminder. Deference to a teaching authority should not be viewed as the cognitive sin it is made out to be, we often do so in other areas of inquiry, e.g., science. Deference might be a very appropriate act of intellectual humility to assent to the moral perceptual abilities of others who lead altruistic lives.

Third, even from a merely human point of view, Catholic teaching has a clarity and thoroughness that should impress even its detractors. While the Church, including its leaders, have made grave moral mistakes, the moral teaching of the Church is actually a light that helps condemn her members' sins, rather than being a result of them. Catholic teaching on healthcare issues is very well-informed and carefully thought through, the result not only of biblical wisdom and ancient tradition but of numerous philosophers, theologians, doctors, and churchmen in dialogue with a full understanding of the relevant science. Even when the voice of the Church is expressed through a single individual—the pope—he never speaks on his own in such matters. One of the reasons that a Magisterium is needed—not merely the Bible or some other holy book—is that technology and other scientific progress is always advancing, sometimes in favor of human dignity, sometimes against it. Only a living teaching authority can keep abreast of it all.

Fourth, also from a human point of view, it is clear that many who have followed the Church's teachings lead flourishing human lives; and this includes ordinary people, extraordinary saints, and medical professionals. Look into the lives of such pioneers of research as Louis Pasteur or Jerome Lejeune, the geneticist who discovered the cause of Down syndrome, among many others. Hopefully, if you are reading this book, it is because you know such witnesses of the joy and love of God in your own lives. Of course, you probably also know people who struggled with some aspect of Catholicism and gave up the faith—and it certainly wouldn't be appropriate to deny the suffering that some have experienced within the Church, especially in situations of abuse. Still, the testimony of those who persevere in seeing the Church's teachings as a gift, not a burden, is that they work; they work to bring the human person into union with the highest goods even in the midst of extreme poverty (Mother Teresa), illness (Damien of Molokai), or political persecution (Thomas More). Conversely, the histories of persons who orient their will around other goods—power, pleasure, or honor—may have plenty of juicy drama, but they lack the peace and experience of lasting relationships with God and others in love of God. If admiration is evidence of a life lived well, then the admiration offered to many who followed the Church's "read" on moral reality would indicate that they had a life lived well.

From a more spiritual point of view, there is still the question for Christians as to why to listen to some man in Rome (to put it crudely) rather than God's voice speaking in their own hearts. It should be noted that the Catholic Church is not against listening for God's voice speaking in one's own heart—in fact, she has many spiritual traditions (such as Ignatian "discernment of spirits") aimed precisely at doing that well! But it is also important to keep in mind the teaching of St. Paul, "For just as the body is one and has many members, and all the members of the body . . . are one body" (1 Cor 12:12). The very idea that God teaches through Revelation to a people—as he does in the Bible—means that we aren't individually on our own to figure everything out through some inner voice. It isn't necessary for each believer to decide on his or her own every aspect of Christian teaching; the teaching instead is given to us as a body of believers that can work together to come to an ever-greater knowledge of God's will.

One might think of the "Magisterium" as a cognitive faculty whose functions are distributed across certain persons (i.e., the college of bishops in union with the Roman Pontiff) and importantly, the Person of the

Holy Spirit. Similar to how different parts of your brain processes visual information (light, shape, contrast, and so on) into a unified perceptual judgment, the Church has different functions distributed across persons and times, and one "function" is the work of the Holy Spirit. Because the faculty includes the executive functioning of God himself, it is by that fact *very* reliable. As Christians, we believe that a good and loving God would not desire to leave his creatures in the dark about how to live flourishing lives. A God who desires loving union with us would not remain forever hidden. As such, it is expected that there would be a *visible* mechanism for teaching us how to realize union with God and love of neighbor. Could God have elected different means by which to renew our moral consciences, such as an invisible and direct enlightenment of our minds? Perhaps, but consider the profusion of cults claiming to function as divine oracles, and how little they agree. Any church or religious community that believes in a personal God has to answer for how there can be a credible, reliable way to know God's teachings amidst this obvious confusion and disagreement. The Catholic Church has a clear answer—the reliability of its teaching office, with many people chosen by Christ working together over time as stewards of his revelation.[17] Our moral cognition needs an outside check on its functioning; one that is visible, verifiable, and has objective markers of reliability noted above. Living one's life in accordance with the Church's moral teachings works in this way. For these reasons, we have cause to trust the "faculty" of the Magisterium as a guide on how best to realize communion with God, ourselves, and fellow persons.

How to Use This Book

The principal aim of this collection is to collate the relevant statements and explanations of the various issues encountered in healthcare delivery and medical research. But more than just providing readers with a one-stop-shop collection, the editors aim to capture something

---

17 The Church's claim of "papal infallibility" does not mean that the pope, and he alone, gets the kind of direct spiritual illumination criticized above. Rather, the grace of teaching authority applies to the *office*, not the individual person *qua* human being. And the office of teaching is ensconced in a network of deliberative processes (e.g., councils, pontifical academies, etc.). If one goal is to create a cooperative community of inquirers, the Holy Spirit is expected to work *through* human beings, not *in spite* of them. Because of this, we should not expect God to have a policy of direct, viz., individualistic, illumination.

more significant: we aim to capture the beauty of the Church's teachings. Quotations were chosen, not just for their length, but also for their way of explaining the Church's understanding on how to love patients. Some of the quotations used may not appear directly relevant to the question but aim to give the reader access to the broader values at stake on some issues (e.g., the section on reproductive technologies). We hope to have captured the beauty of her teachings.

The epistemic reason is, of course, that beauty is a signal for what is true. Sometimes, the beautiful teaching is also the most difficult to realize, for example, the teaching on passive euthanasia for the family that is bedside to their dying loved one who is suffering terminal delirium but is tolerating PEG feeding well. Consider also the military couple trying to conform their marriage to the Church's teachings on responsible parenthood when they can only see each other on rare occasions. To be sure, we do not offer these examples as objections to the Church's teachings, nor that they are inescapably difficult. The point here is only to come clean with the fact that life has its temptations, and these can be different for different people. In those moments, we need a clear view of the Good in our lives in order to make the most loving decision. Apprehending the beauty of what it is to love the human person in these and other circumstances is one means by which we obtain this clearer view.

There are no syllogistic arguments contained herein, no distinctions made at fine-grained detail, no counterexamples, ripostes, and closing repartees. The tone of the presentation is "Look and see. This is the human person, and this is how we believe that we best love him or her." Reflecting on Saint Teresa of Calcutta's work, humanist philosopher Raimond Gaita observes that "her compassion expressed the denial that affliction could ... make a person's life worthless."[18] Suffering does not defile; it does not lessen someone's worth. Saint Teresa of Calcutta's *actions* were meritorious, supererogatory, admirable, and likely issue from good motives or intentions. But what is *beautiful* about her life is that her love reveals the beauty of the lives she loved. "The wonder which is in response to her [Blessed Theresa] is not a wonder at her, but a wonder *that human life could be as her love revealed it to be.*"[19] What Saint Teresa's life shows us is just how valuable those persons are

---

18 Raimond Gaita, *Good and Evil: An Absolute Conception* (New York: Routledge, 2004), 202.

19 Ibid., 205.

around whom their loving activities were oriented. There is a perfect match between her love for the afflicted and their preciousness. Her love reveals to us what might have been obscured otherwise, namely, the depth and comprehensive value "still remaining," if you will, in the afflicted and disabled. Saint Theresa's love reveals that her patients were "fully our equals."[20] Love performs a revelatory role. We do not suppose that reading our volume will give you such a love, but we do hope that we have captured the beauty of the human person in the numerous knotty dimensions of healthcare delivery.

As such, this text can be used by several different groups. Several obvious users include professors who teach healthcare ethics from a religious perspective; patients or their family members who are making decisions and need to understand the general ethical parameters of their decision making; chaplains; and clinicians themselves to better understand their own practice and the wishes of their Catholic patients. As for understanding clinical practice, we think it is not essential that one identify as Christian. The ethical model of healthcare delivery presented in the Church's view is one that can gain acceptance by anyone who adheres to the notion of a natural law inherent in human lives that have intrinsic dignity. Finally, because one goal of this project is to enlighten consciences by capturing the beauty of the Church's teaching, it can be used as a companion piece for retreats.[21]

In using this book, it is important to understand how magisterial documents work, and how they are used here. The questions in this book were prepared by the editors, but the answers are selections that represent some aspects of the Magisterium's authoritative teaching. The Church's teaching function is realized through many different kinds of written documents—encyclical letters, doctrinal definitions, conciliar propositions, guidance documents, answers to *dubia* (questions posed to authorities), and so on. As much as possible, the editors favored writings by those whose teaching function is explicitly a continuation of the apostolic teachers selected by Jesus Christ (i.e., the so-called ordinary and extraordinary Magisterium). Of course, there is variation in how much authority to give these teachings. Teachings enumerated in an encyclical letter, for instance, enjoy greater authority than those enumerated in a

---

20 Ibid., xiii.

21 We would like to thank John M. Haas for conversations spanning several years, the content of which has informed this introduction.

response to *dubia*, or an allocution (papal speech)—unless of course, it is the same teaching that is repeated in each. In this latter case, the teaching gains more authority even if repeated in several answers to *dubia*. Furthermore, it should be mentioned that in some cases, quotations from certain bishops' conferences, or even Catholic bioethical think tanks are used. This is done for one or more of the following reasons: (i) There is no direct teaching on the matter by the Magisterium; (ii) The guidance given reflects the mind of the Church even if not formally taught; (iii) The guidance given is directly relevant and informative. Of course, the more a particular answer relies upon the editors' judgment or less authoritative sources, the more the reader is encouraged to corroborate the guidance with other sources.

Even within very authoritative documents such as an encyclical, or any other Church document, there is variation and room for discernment. One must pay attention to the wording of the teaching, or how forcefully it is stated. A specific example might be to compare Pope St. John Paul II's statements in the encyclical letter *Evangelium vitae* on abortion and the death penalty respectively. Abortion is condemned outright and with no mention of exceptions or conditions, and with no ambiguity of language. Consider the following quotation for illustration.

> Among all the crimes which can be committed against life, procured abortion has characteristics making it particularly serious and deplorable. . . .
>
> The moral gravity of procured abortion is apparent in all its truth if we recognize that we are dealing with murder and, in particular, when we consider the specific elements involved. The one eliminated is a human being at the very beginning of life. No one more absolutely innocent could be imagined. In no way could this human being ever be considered an aggressor, much less an unjust aggressor! He or she is weak, defenseless, even to the point of lacking that minimal form of defense consisting in the poignant power of a newborn baby's cries and tears. The unborn child is totally entrusted to the protection and care of the woman carrying him or her in the womb.[22]

Consider in some contrast, the language used to describe the Church's position on the death penalty.

22 John Paul II, *Evangelium vitae*, 58.

It is clear that, for these purposes to be achieved, the nature and extent of the punishment must be carefully evaluated and decided upon, and ought not go to the extreme of executing the offender except in cases of absolute necessity: in other words, when it would not be possible otherwise to defend society. Today however, as a result of steady improvements in the organization of the penal system, such cases are very rare, if not practically non-existent.[23]

Notice the insertion of an exception, an extreme one, but an exception nonetheless. Notice also the absence of language to the effect that the death penalty as being "deplorable," or "murder." It is certainly true that non-deplorable acts can still be quite immoral and gravely so. The point in contrasting these statements is to highlight the need to exercise discernment even when reading an authoritative document such as a conciliar statement or encyclical letter. One must discern what the teaching is by considering the language used, the conditions enumerated, and the context for the teaching.

Considering the context for a teaching is especially revealing in regard to a topic that had been debated even among ethicists seeking to be faithful to the Church's vision. Pope St. John Paul II offered an allocution on tube feeding patients in a vegetative state. Early in the allocution, the pope makes clear why he is making explicit our duties to all persons.

Faced with patients in ... [a persistent vegetative state], there are some who cast doubt on the persistence of the "human quality" itself, almost as if the adjective "vegetative" (whose use is now solidly established), ... could or should be instead applied to the sick as such.... In this sense, it must be noted that this term, even when confined to the clinical context, is certainly not the most felicitous when applied to human beings. In opposition to such trends of thought, I feel the duty to reaffirm strongly that the intrinsic value and personal dignity of every human being do not change, no matter what the concrete circumstances of his or her life.[24]

---

23 Ibid., 56.

24 John Paul II, Address to the Participants in the International Congress on "Life-sustaining Treatments and Vegetative State: Scientific Advances and Ethical Dilemmas," March 20, 2004, 3.

The context sets the focus of the teaching. In this case, the teaching is meant to enlighten our consciences to the effect that we need to see the inherent dignity of all patients, no matter how grave their disability is. Though specific actions are recommended, i.e., providing such patients with food and water, the teaching is simultaneously meant to correct our moral vision; it aims to correct how we see disabled human life, so that we see patients in such conditions as persons deserving of basic care. Here again, this is not merely a teaching that says, "feed the unconscious," but also it is directing our mind to apprehend the beauty in all human life however disabled or sick.

A final point about discerning the authority of a teaching is to mention the difference between the Church's teachings on faith and morals. Properly understood, much of the Church's moral teaching reflects not simply special religious rules for Catholics, such as the kosher laws of Judaism.[25] Rather, aided by Revelation, she interprets or reads objective moral reality, often referred to as the natural moral law. Just as a scientist interprets data, so too the Church interprets the moral law. For the scientist, the empirical data is a given, with its laws and functions. Moral reality is a given as well. The moral laws or principles of the natural law are guardrails, the following of which contributes to a flourishing life. "But the divine law was given for this chief purpose: so that man might cling to God."[26] The Church does not decide moral reality when a teaching is clarified, rather she reads it, and reports out what it says. In a sense, the Magisterium is an intellectual journalist for moral reality. This is why the Church cannot change her teaching on, for example, contraception. Our task as Catholics is not simply to obey the rules that are thereby formulated, but to look at our particular situation in light of the general rules that we know apply.

In short, to access this collection and explore the beauty and truth found in the Church's teaching, one simply needs to peruse the table of contents, select the questions to which answers are sought, and the richness of magisterial wisdom will be apparent.

---

25 That is to say, moral teaching should be distinguished from disciplines or ritual practices. For example, Eastern Rite Catholics allow priests to marry—under strict conditions—whereas the Roman Rite practices a celibate priesthood. Both practices are, in their respective contexts, reliable *means* to holiness, but they are not different moral judgments. Both practices acknowledge the good of chastity.

26 Thomas Aquinas, *Summa contra gentiles*, bk. 3, 121.1.

Foundational Considerations

Values, Conscience, and Principles

1. What are the fundamental values in light of which the Church assesses bioethical issues?

God's Love for Us

For it is out of goodness--in order to indicate the path of life—that God gives human beings his commandments and the grace to observe them: and it is likewise out of goodness—in order to help them persevere along the same path—that God always offers to everyone his forgiveness.

—Congregation for the Doctrine of the Faith, *Donum vitae*, introduction, 1

The moral life presents itself as the response due to the many gratuitous initiatives taken by God out of love for man.... Thus the moral life, caught up in the gratuitousness of God's love, is called to reflect his glory: "For the one who loves God, it is enough to be pleasing to the One whom he loves: for no greater reward should be sought than that love itself; charity in fact is of God in such a way that God himself is charity."

—John Paul II, *Veritatis splendor*, 10 (quoting Leo the Great, Sermo 92)

The gift of life which God the Creator and Father has entrusted to man calls him to appreciate the inestimable value of what he has been given and to take responsibility for it: this fundamental principle must be placed at the center of one's reflection in order to clarify and solve the moral problems raised by artificial interventions on life.

—Congregation for the Doctrine of the Faith, *Donum vitae*, introduction, 1

The dignity of a person must be recognized in every human being from conception to natural death. This fundamental principle expresses *a great "yes" to human life* and must be at the center of ethical reflection on biomedical research.

—Congregation for the Doctrine of the Faith, *Dignitas personae*, 1

The activity of healthcare workers is basically a service to life and health, which are primary goods of the human person.

—Pontifical Council for Pastoral Assistance to Health Care Workers, *New Charter for Health Care Workers*, 1

The person's right to life—from the moment of his conception till his death—is the first and fundamental right, the root and the source as it were of all other rights. In the same sense, one speaks of the "right to health," that is, to the conditions most favorable for good health.

—John Paul II, Address at the Conclusion of in the Thirty-fifth General Assembly of the World Medical Association, October 29, 1983, 2

Of all visible creatures only man is "able to know and love his creator." He is "the only creature on earth that God has willed for its own sake" and he alone is called to share, by knowledge and love, in God's own life. It was for this end that he was created, and this is the fundamental reason for his dignity.

—*Catechism of the Catholic Church*, 356
(quoting the Vatican Council II,
Gaudium et spes, 12 and 24)

Eternal Calling of the Human Person

Man is called to a fullness of life which far exceeds the dimensions of his earthly existence, because it consists in sharing the very life of God. The loftiness of this supernatural vocation reveals the greatness and inestimable value of human life even in its temporal phase.

—John Paul II, *Evangelium vitae*, 2.

In presenting principles and moral evaluations regarding biomedical research on human life, the Catholic Church draws upon *the light both of reason and of faith* and seeks to set forth an integral vision of man and his vocation, capable of incorporating everything that is good in human activity, as well as in various cultural and religious traditions which not infrequently demonstrate a great reverence for life.

—Congregation for the Doctrine of the Faith, *Dignitas personae*, 3

It is the Church's conviction that what is human is not only received and respected by *faith*, but is also purified, elevated and perfected....

By becoming one of us, the Son makes it possible for us to become "sons of God" (Jn 1:12), "sharers in the divine nature" (2 Pet 1:4)....

The respect for the individual human being, which reason requires, is further enhanced and strengthened in the light of these truths of faith.

—Congregation for the Doctrine of the Faith, *Dignitas personae*, 7

By taking the interrelationship of these two dimensions, *the human and the divine*, as the starting point, one understands better why it is that man has unassailable value: *he possesses an eternal vocation* and *is called to share in the Trinitarian love of the living God.*

This value belongs to all without distinction. By virtue of the simple fact of existing, every human being must be fully respected.

—Congregation for the Doctrine of the Faith, *Dignitas personae*, 8

2. What are the sources of bioethical knowledge?

Conscience is a judgment of reason whereby the human person recognizes the moral quality of a concrete act that he is going to perform, is in the process of performing, or has already completed. In all he says and does, man is obliged to follow faithfully what he knows to be just and right. It is by the judgment of his conscience that man perceives and recognizes the prescriptions of the divine law.

—*Catechism of the Catholic Church*, 1778

On his part, man perceives and acknowledges the imperatives of the divine law through the *mediation of conscience*. In all his activity a man is bound to follow his conscience in order that he may come to God, the end and purpose of life. It follows that he is not to be forced to act in a manner contrary to his conscience.

—Vatican Council II, *Dignitatis humanae*, 3 (emphasis added)

Conscience must be informed, and moral judgment enlightened. A well-formed conscience is upright and truthful. It formulates its judgments according to reason, in conformity with the true good willed by the wisdom of the Creator.

—*Catechism of the Catholic Church*, 1783

3. How does one's conscience become "informed" and "enlightened"?

Then someone came to him and said, "Teacher, what good deed must I do to have eternal life?" And he [Jesus] said to him, ". . . If you wish to enter into life, *keep the commandments. . . .* If you wish to be perfect, go, sell your possessions and give the money to the poor, and you will have treasure in heaven; then come, *follow me.*"

—Matthew 19:16–17, 21 (emphasis added)

People today need to turn to Christ once again in order to receive from him the answer to their questions about what is good and what is evil. Christ is the Teacher, the Risen One who has life in himself and who is always present in his Church and in the world. It is he who opens up to the faithful the book of the Scriptures and, by fully revealing the Father's will, teaches the truth about moral action.

—John Paul II, *Veritatis splendor*, 8, commenting on Matthew 19

4. What role does the Church and magisterial teaching have in forming one's conscience?

The Church has always had the duty of scrutinizing the signs of the times and of interpreting them in the light of the Gospel.

—Vatican Council II, *Gaudium et spes*, 4

The Church's Pastors, in communion with the Successor of Peter, are close to the faithful in this effort [to answer questions on the meaning of life]; they guide and accompany them by their authoritative teaching.

—John Paul II, *Veritatis splendor*, 3

The Church, by expressing an ethical judgment on some developments of recent medical research concerning man and his beginnings, does not intervene in the area proper to medical science itself, but rather calls everyone to ethical and social responsibility for their actions. . . . The intervention of the Magisterium falls within its mission of *contributing to the formation of conscience,* by authentically teaching the truth which is Christ and at the same time by declaring and confirming authoritatively the principles of the moral order which spring from human nature itself.

—Congregation for the Doctrine of the Faith, *Dignitas personae,* 10

In the formation of conscience the Word of God is the light for our path, ... We must also examine our conscience before the Lord's Cross. We are assisted by the gifts of the Holy Spirit, aided by the witness or advice of others and guided by the authoritative teaching of the Church.

—*Catechism of the Catholic Church,* 1785

It is in fact indisputable, as Our predecessors have many times declared, that Jesus Christ, when He communicated His divine power to Peter and the other Apostles and sent them to teach all nations His commandments, constituted them as the authentic guardians and interpreters of the whole moral law, not only, that is, of the law of the Gospel but also of the natural law. For the natural law, too, declares the will of God, and its faithful observance is necessary for men's eternal salvation.

—Paul VI, *Humanae vitae,* 4

5. What is the natural law and what is the divine law?

Natural law is a law accessible to human reason, common to believers and nonbelievers.

—International Theological Commission,
In Search of a Universal Ethic: A New Look at the Natural Law, 34

Foremost in this office comes the natural law which is written and engraved in the soul of each and every man, because it is human reason ordaining him to do good and forbidding him to sin.

—Leo XIII, *Libertas praestantissimum,* 8

The moral law is the work of divine Wisdom. Its biblical meaning can be defined as fatherly instruction, God's pedagogy. It prescribes for man the ways, the rules of conduct, that lead to the promised beatitude.

—*Catechism of the Catholic Church,* 1950

The "divine [eternal] and natural" law shows man the way to follow so as to practice the good and attain his end. The natural law states the first and essential precepts which govern the moral life.... This law is called "natural," not in reference to the nature of irrational beings, but because reason which decrees it properly belongs to human nature.

—*Catechism of the Catholic Church*, 1955

Foremost in this office comes the natural law, which is written and engraved in the mind of every man; and this is nothing but our reason, commanding us to do right and forbidding sin. Nevertheless, all prescriptions of human reason can have force of law only inasmuch as they are the voice and the interpreters of some higher power on which our reason and liberty necessarily depend.... It follows, therefore, that the law of nature [natural law] is the same thing as the eternal law, implanted in rational creatures, and inclining them to their right action and end; and can be nothing else but the eternal reason of God, the Creator and Ruler of all the world.

—Leo XIII, *Libertas praestantissimum*, 8

The highest norm of human life is the divine law—eternal, objective, and universal—whereby God orders, directs, and governs the entire universe and all the ways of the human community by a plan conceived in wisdom and love. Man has been made by God to participate in this law, with the result that, under the gentle disposition of divine Providence, he can come to perceive ever more fully the truth that is unchanging.

—Vatican Council II, *Dignitatis humanae*, 3

Just as in every artificer there pre-exists a type of the things that are made by his art, so too in every governor there must pre-exist the type of the order of those things that are to be done by those who are subject to his government. And just as the type of the things yet to be made by an art is called the art or exemplar of the products of that art, so too the type in him who governs the acts of his subjects, bears the character of a law, ... Now God, by His wisdom, is the Creator of all things in relation to which He stands as the artificer to the products of his art.... Moreover He governs all the acts and movements that are to be found in each single creature, ... Wherefore as the type of the Divine Wisdom, inasmuch as by It all things are created, as the character of art, exemplar or idea; so the type of Divine Wisdom, as moving all things to their due end, bears the character of law. Accordingly the eternal law is nothing else than the type of Divine Wisdom, as directing all actions and movements.

—Thomas Aquinas, *Summa theologiae*, I-II, q. 93, a. 1, resp.

EDITOR'S NOTE: On the use of St. Thomas Aquinas. Pope Pius XII remarks as follows, "If one considers all this well, he will easily see why the Church demands that future priests be instructed in philosophy 'according to the method, doctrine, and principles of the Angelic Doctor [i.e., St. Thomas Aquinas],' since, as we well know from the experience of centuries, the method of Aquinas is singularly preeminent both of teaching students and for bringing truth to light; his doctrine is in harmony with Divine Revelation, and is most effective both for safeguarding the foundation of the faith and for reaping, safely and usefully, the fruits of sound progress." Pope Pius XII, *Humani generis*, 31 (quoting the 1917 *Code of Canon Law*, c. 1366, §2). There is a long tradition in the Catholic Church of studying and following St. Thomas Aquinas's writings. The current 1983 Code of Canon Law, 252, §3, also recommends this as does Leo XIII's 1879 encyclical *Aeterni Patris*. ✢

6. What are the chief moral principles that constitute the natural moral law or serve as the moral guideposts for healthcare decision making?

The Principle of Totality

The principle of totality states that the part exists for the whole, and that consequently the good of the part remains subordinate to the good of the whole; that the whole is decisive for the part and can dispose of it in its own interest.

—Pius XII, "The Moral Limits of Medical Research and Treatment," September 14, 1952

In the absence of other remedies, interventions involving the modification, mutilation, or removal of organs may be necessary to restore the person's health.

The therapeutic manipulation of the human organism is legitimate in this case by virtue of the principle of totality ... , whereby "each particular organ is subordinate to the whole of the body and ought therefore to yield to it, in case of conflict."

—Pontifical Council for Pastoral Assistance to Health Care Workers,
New Charter for Health Care Workers, 88 (quoting Pius XII, Address to
Participants in the Twenty-Sixth Congress of the Italian Urology Association,
October 8, 1953)

Sterilization resulting from a therapeutic act ... [i]s legitimate on the basis of the principle of totality, whereby it is lawful to deprive a person of an organ or of its functioning when it is sick or is the cause of pathological processes that are not otherwise curable. There must also be a foreseeable and reasonable benefit for the patient, and he himself or his legal guardians must have given consent.

—Pontifical Council for Pastoral Assistance to Health Care Workers,
New Charter for Health Care Workers, 20

Since a member is part of the whole human body, it is for the sake of the whole, as the imperfect for the perfect. Hence a member of the human body is to be disposed of according as it is expedient for the body. Now a member of the human body is of itself useful to the good of the whole body, yet, accidentally it may happen to be hurtful, as when a decayed member is a source of corruption to the whole body. Accordingly, so long as a member is healthy and retains its natural disposition, it cannot be cut off without injury to the whole body.

—Thomas Aquinas, *Summa theologiae*, II-II, q. 65, a. 1, resp.

The Principle of Double Effect

Nothing hinders one act from having two effects, only one of which is intended, while the other is beside the intention. *Now moral acts take their species according to what is intended, and not according to what is beside the intention, since this is accidental.* ... Accordingly, the act of self-defense may have two effects, one is the saving of one's life, the other is the slaying of the aggressor. Therefore this act, since one's intention is to save one's own life, is not unlawful, seeing that it is natural to everything to keep itself in "being," as far as possible. And yet, though proceeding from a good intention, an act may be rendered unlawful, if it be out of proportion to the end. Wherefore if a man, in self-defense, uses more than necessary violence, it will be unlawful: whereas if he repel force with moderation his defense will be lawful.

—Thomas Aquinas, *Summa theologiae*, II-II, q. 64, a. 7, resp. (emphasis added)

The Principle of Proportionate Means of Sustaining Life

A person has a moral obligation to use ordinary or proportionate means of preserving his or her life. Proportionate means are those that in the judgment of the patient offer a reasonable hope of benefit and do not entail an excessive burden or impose excessive expense on the family or the community.

—USCCB, *Ethical and Religious Directives for Catholic Health Care Services*, 56

The Principle of Disproportionate Means of Sustaining Life

A person may forgo extraordinary or disproportionate means of preserving life. Disproportionate means are those that in the patient's judgment do not offer a reasonable hope of benefit or entail an excessive burden, or impose excessive expense on the family or the community.

—USCCB, *Ethical and Religious Directives for Catholic Health Care Services*, 57

The Common Good

Every day human interdependence grows more tightly drawn and spreads by degrees over the whole world. As a result the common good, that is, the sum of those conditions of social life which allow social groups and their individual members relatively thorough and ready access to their own fulfillment, today takes on an increasingly universal complexion and consequently involves rights and duties with respect to the whole human race. Every social group must take account of the needs and legitimate aspirations of other groups, and even of the general welfare of the entire human family.

—Vatican Council II, *Gaudium et spes*, 26

First, the common good presupposes *respect for the person* as such. In the name of the common good, public authorities are bound to respect the fundamental and inalienable rights of the human person. Society should permit each of its members to fulfill his vocation. In particular, the common good resides in the conditions for the exercise of the natural freedoms indispensable for the development of the human vocation, such as "the right to act according to a sound norm of conscience and to safeguard ... privacy, and rightful freedom also in matters of religion."

Second, the common good requires the *social well-being* and *development* of the group itself. Development is the epitome of all social duties. Certainly, it is the proper function of authority to arbitrate, in the name of the common good, between various particular interests; but it should make accessible to each what is needed to lead a truly human life: food, clothing, health, work, education and culture, suitable information, the right to establish a family, and so on.

Finally, the common good requires *peace*, that is, the stability and security of a just order. It presupposes that authority should ensure by morally acceptable means the *security* of society and its members. It is the basis of the right to legitimate personal and collective defense.

Each human community possesses a common good which permits it to be recognized as such; it is in the *political community* that its most complete realization is found. It is the role of the State to defend and promote the common good of civil society, its citizens, and intermediate bodies.

Human interdependence is increasing and gradually spreading throughout the world. The unity of the human family, embracing people who enjoy equal natural dignity, implies a *universal common good*. This good calls for an organization of the community of nations able to "provide for the different needs of men; this will involve the sphere of social life to which belong questions of food, hygiene, education, ... and certain situations arising here and there, as for example ... alleviating the miseries of refugees dispersed throughout the world, and assisting migrants and their families."

The common good is always oriented towards the progress of persons: "The order of things must be subordinate to the order of persons, and not the other way around." This order is founded on truth, built up in justice, and animated by love.

—*Catechism of the Catholic Church*, 1907–12,
(quoting Vatican Council II, *Gaudium et spes*, 26 and 84)

Informed Consent

The healthcare worker can intervene if he has previously obtained *the patient's consent, implicitly* (when the medical acts are routine and involve no particular risks) or *explicitly* (in documentable form when the treatments involve risks). Indeed, the healthcare worker has no separate or independent right in dealing with the patient. In general, he can act only if the patient authorizes it explicitly or implicitly (directly or indirectly). Without this authorization, the healthcare worker is arrogating an arbitrary power to himself.

The relationship between the healthcare worker and the patient is a *human relationship of dialogue,* and not a subject–object relation. The patient "is not an anonymous individual" on whom medical expertise is practiced, but "a responsible person, who should be called upon to share in the improvement of his health and in becoming cured. He should be enabled to choose personally, and not be made to submit to the decisions and choices of others."

—Pontifical Council for Pastoral Assistance to Health Care Workers, *New Charter for Health Care Workers,* 96 (quoting John Paul II, Address to the World Congress of Catholic Physicians, October 3, 1982, 4)

On Church Authority

7. What authority does Church teaching have in regard to bioethical issues?

The authority of the Magisterium extends also to the specific precepts of the *natural law,* because their observance, demanded by the Creator, is necessary for salvation.

—*Catechism of the Catholic Church,* 2036

All his [the Christian's] actions, insofar as they are morally either good or bad (that is to say, whether they agree or disagree with the natural and divine law), are subject to the judgment and judicial office of the Church.

—Pius X, *Singulari quadam,* 3

Since, in virtue of her mission received from God, the Church preaches the Gospel to all men and dispenses the treasures of grace, she contributes to the ensuring of peace everywhere on earth and to the placing of the fraternal exchange between men on solid ground *by imparting knowledge of the divine and natural law.*

—Vatican Council II, *Gaudium et spes,* 89 (emphasis added)

It belongs to the Church always and everywhere to announce moral principles, even about the social order, and to render judgment concerning any human affairs insofar as the fundamental rights of the human person or the salvation of souls requires it.

—*Code of Canon Law*, c. 747 §2

The Church's Magisterium does not intervene on the basis of a particular competence in the area of the experimental sciences; but having taken account of the data of research and technology, it intends to put forward, by virtue of its evangelical mission and apostolic duty, the moral teaching corresponding to the dignity of the person and to his or her integral vocation. It intends to do so by expounding the criteria of moral judgment as regards the applications of scientific research and technology, especially in relation to human life and its beginnings. These criteria are the respect, defense, and promotion of man, his "primary and fundamental right" to life, his dignity as a person who is endowed with a spiritual soul and with moral responsibility and who is called to beatific communion with God. The Church's intervention in this field is inspired also by the Love which she owes to man, helping him to recognize and respect his rights and duties.

—Congregation for the Doctrine of the Faith, *Donum vitae*, introduction, 1

8. Why does the Church intervene on bioethical matters?

Today there exists a great multitude of weak and defenseless human beings, unborn children in particular, whose fundamental right to life is being trampled upon. If, at the end of the last century, the Church could not be silent about the injustices of those times, still less can she be silent today, when the social injustices of the past, unfortunately not yet overcome, are being compounded in many regions of the world by still more grievous forms of injustice and oppression, even if these are being presented as elements of progress in view of a new world order.

The present encyclical, ... is therefore meant to be a precise and vigorous reaffirmation of the value of human life and its inviolability, and at the same time a pressing appeal addressed to each and every person, in the name of God: respect, protect, love and serve life, every human life! Only in this direction will you find justice, development, true freedom, peace and happiness!

—John Paul II, *Evangelium vitae*, 5

The Church promotes those aspects of human behavior which favor a true culture of peace, ... The Church renders this service to human society *by preaching the truth about the creation of the world*, which God has placed in human hands so that people may make it fruitful and more perfect through their work; and *by preaching the truth about the Redemption*, whereby the Son of God has saved mankind and at the same time has united all people, making them responsible for one another.

—John Paul II, *Centesimus annus*, 51

The essential meaning of culture consists, ... in the fact that it is a characteristic of human life as such....

Culture is specific way of man's "existing and "being." Man always lives according to a culture which is specifically his, and which, in its turn, creates among men a tie which is also specifically theirs, determining the inter-human and social character of human existence.

—John Paul II, Address to UNESCO:
Man's Entire Humanity Is Expressed in Culture, June 2, 1980, 6

A *new cultural climate* is developing and taking hold, which gives crimes against life a new and ... even more sinister character, giving rise to further grave concern: broad sectors of public opinion justify certain crimes against life [e.g., abortion and euthanasia] in the name of the rights of individual freedom, and on this basis they claim not only exemption from punishment but even authorization by the State, so that these things can be done with total freedom and indeed with the free assistance of healthcare systems.

All this is causing a profound change in the way in which life and relationships between people are considered.... *Choices once unanimously considered criminal and rejected by the common moral sense are gradually becoming socially acceptable.* Even certain sectors of the medical profession, which by its calling is directed to the defense and care of human life, are increasingly willing to carry out these acts against the person. *In this way the very nature of the medical profession is distorted and contradicted*, and the dignity of those who practice it is degraded....

The end result of this is tragic: not only is the fact of the destruction of so many human lives still to be born or in their final stage extremely grave and disturbing, but no less grave and disturbing is the fact that *conscience itself, darkened as it were by such widespread conditioning*, is finding it increasingly difficult to distinguish between good and evil in what concerns the basic value of human life.

—John Paul II, *Evangelium vitae*, 4 (emphasis added)

We are confronted by an even larger reality, which can be described as a veritable structure of sin. This reality is characterized by the emergence of a culture which denies solidarity and, in many cases, takes the form of a veritable "culture of death."

—John Paul II, *Evangelium vitae*, 12

I wish to meditate upon once more and proclaim the Gospel of life, the splendor of truth which *enlightens consciences*, the clear light which corrects the darkened gaze.

—John Paul II, *Evangelium vitae*, 6 (emphasis added)

9. Why does the Church involve herself in healthcare matters?

The Church has always considered serving the sick "an integral part of her mission," combining "the preaching of the Good News with the help and care of the sick."

The vast world of service in response to human suffering "concerns the good of the human person and of society" itself. For this very reason it also poses delicate and unavoidable questions, which involve not only a social and organizational aspect but also a uniquely ethical and religious one. This is because fundamental "human" events are implicated, such as suffering, sickness, and death, together with the related questions about the role of medicine and the mission of physicians with respect to sick persons.

—Pontifical Council for Pastoral Assistance to Health Care Workers,
New Charter for Health Care Workers, preface
(quoting John Paul II, *Dolentium hominum*, 1 and 3)

The Church has always understood herself to be charged by Christ with the care of the poor, the weak, the defenseless, the suffering and those who mourn. This means that, as you alleviate suffering and seek to heal, you also bear witness to the Christian view of suffering and to the meaning of life and death as taught by your Christian faith.

In the complex world of modern health care in industrialized society, this witness must be given in a variety of ways. First, it requires continual efforts *to ensure that everyone has access to health care.* . . . In seeking to treat patients equally, *regardless of social and economic status,* you proclaim to your fellow citizens and to the world Christ's special love for the neglected and powerless. This particular challenge is a consequence of your Christian dedication and conviction, and it calls for great courage on the part of Catholic bodies and institutions operating in the field of health care.

Similarly, the love with which Catholic health care is performed and its professional excellence have the value of a sign testifying to the Christian view of the human person. *The inalienable dignity of every human being is, of course, fundamental to all Catholic health care.* All who come to you for help are worthy of respect and love, for all have been created in the image and likeness of God. All have been redeemed by Christ and, in their sufferings, bear his Cross.

The structural changes which have been taking place within Catholic health care in recent years have increased the challenge of *preserving and even strengthening the Catholic identity of the institutions and the spiritual quality of the services given.* The presence of dedicated women and men religious in hospitals and nursing homes has ensured in the past, and continues to ensure in the present, that spiritual dimension so characteristic of Catholic healthcare centers. The reduced number of religious and new forms of ownership and management should not lead to a loss of a spiritual atmosphere, or to a loss of a sense of vocation in caring for the sick. This is an area in which the Catholic laity, at all levels of health care, have an opportunity to manifest the depth of their faith and to play their own specific part in the Church's mission of evangelization and service.

... Catholic health care must always be carried out within the framework of the Church's saving mission. This mission she has received from her divine Founder, and she has accomplished it down through the ages with the help of the Holy Spirit who guides her into the fullness of truth. *Your ministry therefore must also reflect the mission of the Church as the teacher of moral truth,* ...

Many times in recent years the Church has addressed issues related to the advances of biomedical technology. She does so not in order to discourage scientific progress or to judge harshly those who seek to extend the frontiers of human knowledge and skill, but in order to affirm the moral truths which must guide the application of this knowledge and skill. Ultimately, the purpose of the Church's teaching in this field is *to defend the innate dignity and fundamental rights of the human person.*

—John Paul II, Address to the Leaders
in Catholic Health Care, September 14, 1987, 3–4

10. What role does the Church play in health care?

The deep interest which the Church has always demonstrated for the world of the suffering is well known. In this for that matter, she has done nothing more than follow the very eloquent example of her Founder and Master. In the apostolic letter *Salvifici doloris* of February 11, 1984, I emphasized that "in his messianic activity in the midst of Israel, Christ drew increasingly closer *to the world of human suffering.* 'He went about doing good,' and his actions concerned primarily those who were suffering and seeking help."

In fact, over the course of the centuries the Church has felt strongly that service to the sick and suffering is an integral part of her mission, and not only has she encouraged among Christians the blossoming of various works of mercy, but she has also established many religious institutions within her with the specific aim to fostering, organizing, improving and increasing help to the sick. Missionaries, on their part, in carrying out the work of evangelization have constantly combined the preaching of the Good News with the help and care of the sick.

In her approach to the sick and to the mystery of suffering, the Church is guided [by] a precise concept of the human person and of his destiny in God's plan. She holds that medicine and therapeutic cures be directed not only to the good and the health of the body, but to the person as such who, in his body, is stricken by evil. In fact, illness and suffering are not experiences which concern only man's physical substance, but man in his entirety and in his somatic-spiritual unity. For that matter, it is known how often the illness which is manifested in the body has its origins and its true cause in the recesses of the human psyche.

Illness and suffering are phenomena which, if examined in depth, always pose questions which go beyond medicine itself to touch the essence of the human condition in this world. Therefore, it is easy to understand the importance, in the social-healthcare services of the presence not only of pastors of souls, but also of workers who are led by an integrally human view of illness and who as a result are able to effect a fully human approach to [the] sick parson who is suffering. For the Christian, Christ's redemption and his salvific grace reach the whole man in his human condition and therefore reach also illness, suffering, and death.

—John Paul II, *Dolentium hominum*, 1–2

From century to century the Christian community in revealing and communicating its healing love and the consolation of Jesus Christ has reenacted the gospel parable of the Good Samaritan in caring for the vast multitude of persons who are sick and suffering. This came about through the untiring commitment of all those who have taken care of the sick and suffering as a result of science and the medical arts as well as the skilled and generous service of healthcare workers. Today there is an increase in the presence of lay women and men in Catholic hospital[s] and healthcare institutions. At times the lay faithful's presence in these institutions is total and exclusive. It is to just such people—doctors, nurses, other healthcare workers, volunteers—that the call becomes the living sign of Jesus Christ and his Church in showing love towards the sick and suffering.

—John Paul II, *Christifideles laici*, 53

About the Human Person, Suffering, and Evil

11. What does the Church teach about the human person?

The human person, created in the image of God, is a being at once corporeal and spiritual. The biblical account expresses this reality in symbolic language when it affirms that "then the LORD God formed man of dust from the ground, and breathed into his nostrils the breath of life; and man became a living being" (Gn 2:7). Man, whole and entire, is therefore willed by God.

In Sacred Scripture the term "soul" often refers to human *life* or the entire human *person*. But "soul" also refers to the innermost aspect of man, that which is of greatest value in him, that by which he is most especially in God's image: "soul" signifies the *spiritual principle* in man.

The human body shares in the dignity of "the image of God": it is a human body precisely because it is animated by a spiritual soul, and it is the whole human person that is intended to become, in the body of Christ, a temple of the Spirit: (1 Cor 6:19–20; 15:44–45) "Man, though made of body and soul, is a unity. Through his very bodily condition he sums up in himself the elements of the material world. Through him they are thus brought to their highest perfection and can raise their voice in praise freely given to the Creator. For this reason man may not despise his bodily life. Rather he is obliged to regard his body as good and to hold it in honor since God has created it and will raise it up on the last day"

The unity of soul and body is so profound that one has to consider the soul to be the "form" of the body: i.e., it is because of its spiritual soul that the body made of matter becomes a living, human body; spirit and

37

matter, in man, are not two natures united, but rather their union forms a single nature.

The Church teaches that every spiritual soul is created immediately by God—it is not "produced" by the parents—and also that it is immortal: it does not perish when it separates from the body at death, and it will be reunited with the body at the final Resurrection.

—*Catechism of the Catholic Church*, 362–66
(quoting Vatican Council II, *Gaudium et spes*, 14)

God, who has fatherly concern for everyone, has willed that all men should constitute one family and treat one another in a spirit of brotherhood. For having been created in the image of God, who "from one man has created the whole human race and made them live all over the face of the earth" (Acts 17:26), all men are called to one and the same goal, namely God Himself.

For this reason, love for God and neighbor is the first and greatest commandment. Sacred Scripture, however, teaches us that the love of God cannot be separated from love of neighbor: "If there is any other commandment, it is summed up in this saying: Thou shalt love thy neighbor as thyself.... Love therefore is the fulfillment of the Law" (Rom 13:9–10). To men growing daily more dependent on one another, and to a world becoming more unified every day, this truth proves to be of paramount importance.

Indeed, the Lord Jesus, when He prayed to the Father, "that all may be one ... as we are one" (Jn 17:21–22) opened up vistas closed to human reason, for He implied a certain likeness between the union of the divine Persons, and the unity of God's sons in truth and charity. This likeness reveals that man, who is the only creature on earth which God willed for itself, cannot fully find himself except through a sincere gift of himself.

—Vatican Council II, *Gaudium et spes*, 24

Man cannot live without love. He remains a being that is incomprehensible for himself, his life is senseless, if love is not revealed to him, if he does not encounter love, if he does not experience it and make it his own, if he does not participate intimately in it. This, as has already been said, is why Christ the Redeemer "fully reveals man to himself." If we may use the expression, this is the human dimension of the mystery of the Redemption. In this dimension man finds again the greatness, dignity, and value that belong to his humanity. In the mystery of the Redemption man becomes newly "expressed" and, in a way, is newly created. He is newly created! "There is neither Jew nor Greek, there is neither slave nor free, there is neither male nor female; for you are all one in Christ Jesus" (Gal 3:28). The man who wishes to understand himself thoroughly—and not just in accordance with immediate, partial, often superficial, and even illusory standards and measures of his being—he must with his unrest, uncertainty, and even his weakness and sinfulness, with his life and death, draw near to Christ. He must, so to speak, enter into him with all his own self, he must "appropriate" and assimilate the whole of the reality of the Incarnation and Redemption in order to find himself. If this profound process takes place within him, he then bears fruit not only of adoration of God but also of deep wonder at himself. How precious must man be in the eyes of the Creator, if he "gained so great a Redeemer," and if God "gave his only Son" in order that man "should not perish but have eternal life" (Jn 3:16).

—John Paul II, *Redemptor hominis*, 10 (quoting Vatican Council II, *Gaudium et spes*, 22; and the *Exsultet* at the Easter Vigil)

12. How might suffering be viewed in the world?

In order to perceive the true answer to the "why" of suffering, we must look to the revelation of divine love, the ultimate source of the meaning of everything that exists. Love is also the richest source of the meaning of suffering, which always remains a mystery: we are conscious of the insufficiency and inadequacy of our explanations. Christ causes us to enter into the mystery and to discover the "why" of suffering, as far as we are capable of grasping the sublimity of divine love.

In order to discover the profound meaning of suffering, following the revealed word of God, we must open ourselves wide to the human subject in his manifold potentiality. We must above all accept the light of Revelation not only insofar as it expresses the transcendent order of justice but also insofar as it illuminates this order with Love, as the definitive source of everything that exists. Love is: also the fullest source of the answer to the question of the meaning of suffering. This answer has been given by God to man in the Cross of Jesus Christ.

—John Paul II, *Salvifici doloris*, 13

Down through the centuries and generations it has been seen that *in suffering there is concealed* a particular *power that draws a person interiorly close to Christ*, a special grace. To this grace many saints, such as Saint Francis of Assisi, Saint Ignatius of Loyola, and others, owe their profound conversion. A result of such a conversion is not only that the individual discovers the salvific meaning of suffering but above all that he becomes a completely new person. He discovers a new dimension, as it were, of *his entire life and vocation*. This discovery is a particular confirmation of the spiritual greatness which in man surpasses the body in a way that is completely beyond compare. When this body is gravely ill, totally incapacitated, and the person is almost incapable of living and acting, all the more do interior *maturity and spiritual greatness* become evident, constituting a touching lesson to those who are healthy and normal.

—John Paul II, *Salvifici doloris*, 26

Following the parable of the Gospel, we could say that suffering, which is present under so many different forms in our human world, is also present in order *to unleash love in the human person*, that unselfish gift of one's "I" on behalf of other people, especially those who suffer. The world of human suffering unceasingly calls for, so to speak, another world: the world of human love; and in a certain sense man owes to suffering that unselfish love which stirs in his heart and actions. The person who is a " neighbor" cannot indifferently pass by the suffering of another: this in the name of fundamental human solidarity, still more in the name of love of neighbor. He must "stop," "sympathize," just like the Samaritan of the Gospel parable. The parable in itself expresses *a deeply Christian truth*, but one that at the same time is very universally human. It is not without reason that, also in ordinary speech, any activity on behalf of the suffering and needy is called "Good Samaritan" work.

—John Paul II, *Salvifici doloris*, 29

Human Sickness and Its Meaning in the Mystery of Salvation

Suffering and illness have always been among the greatest problems that trouble the human spirit. Christians feel and experience pain as do all other people; yet their faith helps them to grasp more deeply the mystery of suffering and to bear their pain with greater courage. From Christ's words they know that sickness has meaning and value for their own salvation and for the salvation of the world. They also know that Christ, who during his life often visited and healed the sick, loves them in their illness.

Although closely linked with the human condition, sickness cannot as a general rule be regarded as a punishment inflicted on each individual for personal sins (see Jn 9:3). Christ himself, who is without sin, in fulfilling the words of Isaiah took on all the wounds of his passion and shared in all human pain (see Is 53:4–5). Christ is still pained and tormented in his members, made like him. Still, our afflictions seem but momentary and slight when compared to the greatness of the eternal glory for which they prepare us (see 2 Cor 4:17).

Part of the plan laid out by God's providence is that we should fight strenuously against all sickness and carefully seek the blessings of good health, so that we may fulfill our role in human society and in the Church. Yet we should always be prepared to fill up what is lacking in Christ's suffering for the salvation of the world as we look forward to creation's being set free in the glory of the children of God (see Col 1:24; Rom 8:19–21). Moreover, the role of the sick in the Church is to be a reminder to others of the essential or higher things. By their witness the sick show that our mortal life must be redeemed through the mystery of Christ's death and resurrection.

The sick person is not the only one who should fight against illness. Doctors and all who are devoted in any way to caring for the sick should consider it their duty to use all the means which in their judgment may help the sick, both physically and spiritually. In so doing, they are fulfilling the command of Christ to visit the sick, for Christ implied that those who visit the sick should be concerned for the whole person and offer both physical relief and spiritual comfort.

—*Pastoral Care of the Sick: Rites of Anointing and Viaticum,*
general introduction, 1–4

13. What is meant by "intrinsic evil"?

Reason attests that there are objects of the human act which are by their nature "incapable of being ordered" to God, because they radically contradict the good of the person made in his image. These are the acts which, in the Church's moral tradition, have been termed "intrinsically evil" (*intrinsece malum*): they are such *always and per se,* in other words, on account of their very object, and quite apart from the ulterior intentions of the one acting and the circumstances. Consequently, without in the least denying the influence on morality exercised by circumstances and especially by intentions, the Church teaches that "there exist acts which *per se* and in themselves, independently of circumstances, are always seriously wrong by reason of their object." The Second Vatican Council itself, in discussing the respect due to the human person, gives a number of examples of such acts: "Whatever is hostile to life itself, such

41

as any kind of homicide, genocide, abortion, euthanasia and voluntary suicide; whatever violates the integrity of the human person, such as mutilation, physical and mental torture and attempts to coerce the spirit; whatever is offensive to human dignity, such as subhuman living conditions, arbitrary imprisonment, deportation, slavery, prostitution and trafficking in women and children; degrading conditions of work which treat laborers as mere instruments of profit, and not as free responsible persons: all these and the like are a disgrace, and so long as they infect human civilization they contaminate those who inflict them more than those who suffer injustice, and they are a negation of the honor due to the Creator."

With regard to intrinsically evil acts, and in reference to contraceptive practices whereby the conjugal act is intentionally rendered infertile, Pope Paul VI teaches: "Though it is true that sometimes it is lawful to tolerate a lesser moral evil in order to avoid a greater evil or in order to promote a greater good, it is never lawful, even for the gravest reasons, to do evil that good may come of it (cf. Rom 3:8)—in other words, to intend directly something which of its very nature contradicts the moral order, and which must therefore be judged unworthy of man, even though the intention is to protect or promote the welfare of an individual, of a family, or of society in genera."

In teaching the existence of intrinsically evil acts, the Church accepts the teaching of Sacred Scripture. The Apostle Paul emphatically states: "Do not be deceived: neither the immoral, nor idolaters, nor adulterers, nor sexual perverts, nor thieves, nor the greedy, nor drunkards, nor revilers, nor robbers will inherit the Kingdom of God" (1 Cor 6:9–10).

If acts are intrinsically evil, a good intention or particular circumstances can diminish their evil, but they cannot remove it. They remain "irremediable" evil acts; per se and in themselves they are not capable of being ordered to God and to the good of the person. "As for acts which are themselves sins (cum iam opera ipsa peccata sunt)," Saint Augustine writes, "like theft, fornication, blasphemy, who would dare affirm that, by doing them for good motives (causis bonis), they would no longer be sins, or, what is even more absurd, that they would be sins that are justified."

Consequently, circumstances or intentions can never transform an act intrinsically evil by virtue of its object into an act "subjectively" good or defensible as a choice.

Furthermore, an intention is good when it has as its aim the true good of the person in view of his ultimate end. But acts whose object is "not capable of being ordered" to God and "unworthy of the human person" are always and in every case in conflict with that good. Consequently, respect for norms which prohibit such acts and oblige *semper et pro semper*, that is, without any exception, not only does not inhibit a good intention, but actually represents its basic expression.

The doctrine of the object as a source of morality represents an authentic explication of the biblical morality of the Covenant and of the commandments, of charity and of the virtues. The moral quality of human acting is dependent on this fidelity to the commandments, as an expression of obedience and of love. For this reason—we repeat—the opinion must be rejected as erroneous which maintains that it is impossible to qualify as morally evil according to its species the deliberate choice of certain kinds of behavior or specific acts, without taking into account the intention for which the choice was made or the totality of the foreseeable consequences of that act for all persons concerned. Without the *rational determination of the morality of human acting* as stated above, it would be impossible to affirm the existence of an "objective moral order" and to establish any particular norm the content of which would be binding without exception. This would be to the detriment of human fraternity and the truth about the good, and would be injurious to ecclesial communion as well.

—John Paul II, *Veritatis splendor*, 80–82
(quoting John Paul II, *Reconciliatio et Paenitentia*, 17; Vatican Council II,
Gaudium et spes, 27; Paul VI, *Humanae vitae*, 14; Augustine, *Contra Mendacium*)

Loving Ourselves and Others

14. Is there a moral obligation for a person to care for his- or herself?

Preventing is better than treating, both because it spares the person the discomfort and suffering of illness, and also because it spares society the costs of treatment, which are not just economic.

—Pontifical Council for Pastoral Assistance to Health Care Workers,
New Charter for Health Care Workers, 67

Life and physical health are precious gifts entrusted to us by God. We must take reasonable care of them, taking into account the needs of others and the common good.

—*Catechism of the Catholic Church*, 2288

15. Do we have an obligation to exercise or otherwise improve or maintain our health status?

As individuals we show respect for our own life and dignity when we adopt lifestyles that enhance our health and well-being.

—USCCB, *Health and Health Care*, III, A

16. Do we have an obligation to avoid drug, tobacco (i.e., nicotine), or alcohol dependency?

EDITOR'S NOTE: Drug dependence varies in *degrees* from intermittent tobacco use to heroin addiction. But The Church's moral guidance on this issue refers to action *types or kinds*, namely, *dependency* on drugs. Dependency in this context refers to the will's orientation towards repeatedly using that which is to some extent harmful to the person's health and well-being. ✣

[Drug abuse] is always illicit, because it implies an unjustified and irrational refusal to think, will, and act as free persons.

—John Paul II, Address to the Participants in the Sixth International Conference on Drugs and Alcohol, November 23, 1991, 4

The *use of drugs* inflicts very grave damage on human health and life. Their use, except on strictly therapeutic grounds, is a grave offense. Clandestine production of and trafficking in drugs are scandalous practices. They constitute direct co-operation in evil, since they encourage people to practices gravely contrary to the moral law.

—*Catechism of the Catholic Church*, 2291

At the root of alcohol and drug abuse—taking into account the painful complexity of causes and situations—there is usually an existential vacuum, due to an absence of values and a lack of self-esteem, of trust in others and in life in general.

—John Paul II, Address to the Participants in the Sixth International Conference on Drugs and Alcohol, November 23, 1991, 2

17. What distinctive ethical principles should Catholic healthcare workers bear in mind when treating patients with drug, tobacco, or alcohol dependencies?

The new forms of slavery to drugs and the lack of hope into which so many people fall can be explained not only in sociological and psychological terms but also in essentially spiritual terms. The emptiness in which the soul feels abandoned, despite the availability of countless therapies for body and psyche, leads to suffering. *There cannot be holistic development and universal common good unless people's spiritual and moral welfare is taken into account*, considered in their totality as body and soul.

—Benedict XVI, *Caritas in veritate*, 76

If . . . a direct appeal is made to his [a person's] instincts—while ignoring in various ways the reality of the person as intelligent and free—then *consumer attitudes* and *life-styles* can be created which are objectively improper and often damaging to his physical and spiritual health. . . .

A striking example of artificial consumption contrary to the health and dignity of the human person, and certainly not easy to control, is the use of drugs. Widespread drug use is a sign of a serious malfunction in the social system; it also implies a materialistic and, in a certain sense, destructive "reading" of human needs. In this way the innovative capacity of a free economy is brought to a one-sided and inadequate conclusion. Drugs, as well as pornography and other forms of consumerism which exploit the frailty of the weak, tend to fill the resulting spiritual void.

—John Paul II, *Centesimus annus*, 36

2

At the Beginning of Life

Loving the Pre-born

18. Why is abortion immoral? Isn't this just a religious teaching that applies only to Catholics?

> You shall not murder a child by abortion nor kill that which is born.
>
> —*Didache*, 2

> The inviolability of the human person from the moment of conception forbids abortion, which is the destruction of prenatal life and a direct violation of the human being's fundamental right to life.
>
> —Pontifical Council for Pastoral Assistance to Health Care Workers,
> *New Charter for Health Care Workers*, 51

> The body of a human being, from the very first stages of its existence, can never be reduced merely to a group of cells. The embryonic human body develops progressively according to a well-defined program with its proper finality, as is apparent in the birth of every baby.
>
> —Congregation for the Doctrine of the Faith, *Dignitas personae*, 4

> *The human being is to be respected and treated as a person from the moment of conception*; and therefore from that same moment his rights as a person must be recognized, among which in the first place is the inviolable right of every innocent human being to life.
>
> —Congregation for the Doctrine of the Faith, *Donum vitae*, I.1

Direct abortion, that is, abortion willed as an end or as a means, always constitutes a grave moral disorder, since it is the deliberate killing of an innocent human being....

No circumstance, no purpose, no law whatsoever can ever make licit an act which is intrinsically illicit, since it is contrary to the Law of God which is written in every human heart, knowable by reason itself, and proclaimed by the Church.

—John Paul II, *Evangelium vitae*, 62

The findings of human biology confirm that "in the zygote resulting from fertilization the biological identity of a new human individual is already constituted." This is the individuality belonging to a being that is autonomous, intrinsically determined, and self-realizing with gradual continuity.

—Pontifical Council for Pastoral Assistance to Health Care Workers,
New Charter for Health Care Workers, 40 (quoting Congregation
for the Doctrine of the Faith, *Donum vitae*, I.1)

From the time that the ovum is fertilized, a life is begun which is neither that of the father nor of the mother, it is rather the life of a new human being with his own growth. It would never be made human if it were not human already.

To this perpetual evidence—perfectly independent of the discussions on the moment of animation—modern genetic science brings valuable confirmation. It has demonstrated that, from the first instant, there is established the program of what this living being will be: a man, this individual man with his characteristic aspects already well determined. Right from fertilization is begun the adventure of a human life, and each of its capacities requires time—a rather lengthy time—to find its place and to be in a position to act.

—Congregation for the Doctrine of the Faith,
Declaration on Procured Abortion, 13

The first right of the human person is his life. He has other goods, and some are more precious; but this one is fundamental—the condition of all the others. Hence it must be protected above all others. It does not belong to society, nor does it belong to public authority in any form to recognize this right for some and not for others: all discrimination is evil, whether it be founded on race, sex, color, or religion. It is not recognition by another that constitutes this right. This right is antecedent to its recognition; it demands recognition, and it is strictly unjust to refuse it.

—Congregation for the Doctrine of the Faith,
Declaration on Procured Abortion, 11

19. On what authority does the Church speak on the issue of abortion?

The Church is too conscious of the fact that it belongs to her vocation to defend man against everything that could disintegrate or lessen his dignity to remain silent on such a topic. Because the Son of God became man, there is no man who is not His brother in humanity and who is not called to become a Christian in order to receive salvation from Him.

—Congregation for the Doctrine of the Faith,
Declaration on Procured Abortion, 1

20. Shouldn't the choice about abortion be allowed anyway since people disagree on its moral status?

Ethical pluralism is claimed to be a normal consequence of ideological pluralism. There is, however, a great difference between the one and the other, for action affects the interests of others more quickly than does mere opinion. Moreover, one can never claim freedom of opinion as a pretext for attacking the rights of others, most especially the right to life.

—Congregation for the Doctrine of the Faith,
Declaration on Procured Abortion, 2

21. Is there a specifically religious idea that argues against abortion?

Certainly God has created beings who have only one lifetime, and physical death cannot be absent from the world of those with a bodily existence. But what is immediately willed is life, and in the visible universe everything has been made for man, who is the image of God and the world's crowning glory.

—Congregation for the Doctrine of the Faith,
Declaration on Procured Abortion, 5

22. Is an abortion very early on in human development permissible?

EDITOR'S NOTE: This question is addressing the position of "delayed ensoulment" according to which the soul is not infused by God until the human conceptus develops the type of "material" able to receive the rational soul, namely, a rudimentary brain. The idea is that an abortion prior to ensoulment does not kill a person. The following quotations address this idea. ✢

It [newly conceived life] would never be made human if it were not human already.

—Congregation for the Doctrine of the Faith,
Declaration on Procured Abortion, 12

Although the presence of the spiritual soul cannot be observed experimentally, the conclusions of science regarding the human embryo give "a valuable indication for discerning by the use of reason a personal presence at the moment of the first appearance of a human life: how could a human individual not be a human person?" Indeed, the reality of the human being for the entire span of life, both before and after birth, does not allow us to posit either a change in nature or a gradation in moral value, since it possesses *full anthropological and ethical status*. The human embryo has, therefore, from the very beginning, the dignity proper to a person.

—Congregation for the Doctrine of the Faith, *Dignitas personae*, 5
(quoting Congregation for the Doctrine of the Faith, *Donum vitae*, I.1)

In the course of history, the Fathers of the Church, her Pastors, and her Doctors have taught the same doctrine—the various opinions on the infusion of the spiritual soul did not introduce any doubt about the illicitness of abortion. ... The first Council of Mainz in 847 reconsidered the penalties against abortion which had been established by preceding councils. It decided that the most rigorous penance would be imposed "on women who procure the elimination of the fruit conceived in their womb." The Decree of Gratian reported the following words of Pope Stephen V: "That person is a murderer who causes to perish by abortion what has been conceived." St. Thomas, the Common Doctor of the Church, teaches that abortion is a grave sin against the natural law. At the time of the Renaissance, Pope Sixtus V condemned abortion with the greatest severity. A century later, Innocent XI rejected the propositions of certain lax canonists who sought to excuse an abortion procured before the moment accepted by some as the moment of the spiritual animation of the new being.

—Congregation for the Doctrine of the Faith,
Declaration on Procured Abortion, 7

23. Is a direct abortion in the cases of disability or certain death of the baby soon after birth, such as in the case of anencephaly, permissible?

Abortion (that is, the directly intended termination of pregnancy before viability or the directly intended destruction of a viable fetus) is never permitted. Every procedure whose sole immediate effect is the termination of pregnancy before viability is an abortion, which, in its moral context, includes the interval between conception and implantation of the embryo.

—USCCB, *Ethical and Religious Directives
for Catholic Health Care Services,* 45

Operations, treatments, and medications that have as their direct purpose the cure of a proportionately serious pathological condition of a pregnant woman are permitted when they cannot be safely postponed until the unborn child is viable, even if they will result in the death of the unborn child.

—USCCB, *Ethical and Religious Directives
for Catholic Health Care Services,* 47

It is clear that before "viability" it is never permitted to terminate the gestation of an anencephalic child as the *means* of avoiding psychological or physical risks to the mother. Nor is such termination permitted after "viability" if early delivery endangers the child's life due to complications of prematurity. In such cases, it cannot reasonably be maintained that such a termination is simply a side effect of the treatment of a pathology of the mother (as described in Directive 47). Anencephaly is not a pathology of the mother, but of the child, and terminating her pregnancy cannot be a treatment of a pathology she does not have. Only if the complications of the pregnancy result in a life-threatening pathology of the mother, may the treatment of this pathology be permitted even at a risk to the child, and then only if the child's death is not a means to treating the mother.

—USCCB, *Moral Principles Concerning Infants with Anencephaly*, September 19, 1996

24. Are not the negative consequences of restricting access to abortion such as the child living in poverty, or that she or he lives with a mental disability, cases of rape arguments for abortion's permissibility?

We proclaim only that none of these reasons can ever objectively confer the right to dispose of another's life, even when that life is only beginning. With regard to the future unhappiness of the child, no one, not even the father or mother, can act as its substitute—even if it is still in the embryonic stage—to choose in the child's name, life or death. The child itself, when grown up, will never have the right to choose suicide; no more may his parents choose death for the child while it is not of an age to decide for itself. Life is too fundamental a value to be weighed against even very serious disadvantages.

—Congregation for the Doctrine of the Faith, *Declaration on Procured Abortion*, 14

Never, under any pretext, may abortion be resorted to, either by a family or by the political authority, as a legitimate means of regulating births. The damage to moral values is always a greater evil for the common good than any disadvantage in the economic or demographic order.

—Congregation for the Doctrine of the Faith, *Declaration on Procured Abortion*, 18

25. Does not women's emancipation depend upon access to abortion? Isn't sexual freedom a value that is hindered by having direct abortion illegal?

The movement for the emancipation of women, insofar as it seeks essentially to free them from all unjust discrimination, is on perfectly sound ground. In the different forms of cultural background there is a great deal to be done in this regard. But one cannot change nature. Nor can one exempt women, any more than men, from what nature demands of them. Furthermore, all publicly recognized freedom is always limited by the certain rights of others.

The same must be said of the claim to sexual freedom. If by this expression one is to understand the mastery progressively acquired by reason and by authentic love over instinctive impulse, without diminishing pleasure but keeping it in its proper place—and in this sphere this is the only authentic freedom—then there is nothing to object to. But this kind of freedom will always be careful not to violate justice. If, on the contrary, one is to understand that men and women are "free" to seek sexual pleasure to the point of satiety, without taking into account any law or the essential orientation of sexual life to its fruits of fertility, then this idea has nothing Christian in it. It is even unworthy of man. In any case it does not confer any right to dispose of human life—even if embryonic—or to suppress it on the pretext that it is burdensome.

—Congregation for the Doctrine of the Faith,
Declaration on Procured Abortion, 15–16

In this regard the [Second Vatican] Council declares that the moral goodness of the acts proper to conjugal life, acts which are ordered according to true human dignity, "does not depend solely on sincere intentions or on an evaluation of motives. It must be determined by objective standards. These, based on the nature of the human person and his acts, preserve the full sense of mutual self-giving and human procreation in the context of true love."

These final words briefly sum up the Council's teaching ... on the finality of the sexual act and on the principal criterion of its morality: it is respect for its finality that ensures the moral goodness of this act.

—Congregation for the Doctrine of the Faith, *Persona humana*, V (quoting
Vatican Council II, *Gaudium et spes*, 51)

Motherhood *in the bio-physical sense* appears to be passive: the formation process of a new life "takes place" in her, in her body, which is nevertheless profoundly involved in that process. At the same time, motherhood *in its personal-ethical sense* expresses a very important creativity on the part of the woman, upon whom the very humanity of the new human being mainly depends. In this sense too the woman's motherhood presents a special call and a special challenge to the man and to his fatherhood.

The biblical exemplar of the "woman" finds its culmination *in the motherhood of the Mother of God*.... We see that through Mary—through her maternal "fiat," ("Let it be done to me")—God *begins a New Covenant with humanity*.... Precisely because this Covenant is to be fulfilled "in flesh and blood," its beginning is in the Mother. Thanks solely to her and to her virginal and maternal "fiat," the "Son of the Most High" can say to the Father: "A body you have prepared for me. Lo, I have come to do your will, O God" (cf. Heb 10:5, 7).

Motherhood has been introduced into the order of the Covenant that God made with humanity in Jesus Christ. *Each and every time that motherhood is repeated in human history, it is always related to the Covenant which God established with the human race through the motherhood of the Mother of God* [emphasis added].

—John Paul II, *Mulieris dignitatem*, 19

26. What about the fact that there are a plurality of opinions on the issue, or that abortion will occur anyway even if it is illegal, or that it would be impossible to punish all of those who break the law?

These arguments and others in addition that are heard from varying quarters are not conclusive. It is true that civil law cannot expect to cover the whole field of morality or to punish all faults. No one expects it to do so. It must often tolerate what is in fact a lesser evil, in order to avoid a greater one. One must, however, be attentive to what a change in legislation can represent. Many will take as authorization what is perhaps only the abstention from punishment. Even more, in the present case, this very renunciation seems at the very least to admit that the legislator no longer considers abortion a crime against human life, since murder is still always severely punished. It is true that it is not the task of the law to choose between points of view or to impose one rather than another. But the life of the child takes precedence over all opinions. One cannot invoke freedom of thought to destroy this life.

—Congregation for the Doctrine of the Faith, *Declaration on Procured Abortion*, 20

It is at all times the task of the State to preserve each person's rights and to protect the weakest. In order to do so the State will have to right many wrongs. The law ... cannot act contrary to a law which is deeper and more majestic than any human law: the natural law engraved in men's hearts by the Creator as a norm which reason clarifies and strives to formulate properly, and which one must always struggle to understand better, but which it is always wrong to contradict. Human law can abstain from punishment, but it cannot declare to be right what would be opposed to the natural law.

—Congregation for the Doctrine of the Faith,
Declaration on Procured Abortion, 21

27. Is it permissible to cooperate in an abortion either as a clinician or a citizen who is voting for certain policies?

It must in any case be clearly understood that whatever may be laid down by civil law in this matter, man can never obey a law which is in itself immoral, and such is the case of a law which would admit in principle the liceity of abortion. Nor can he take part in a propaganda campaign in favor of such a law, or vote for it. Moreover, he may not collaborate in its application. It is, for instance, inadmissible that doctors or nurses should find themselves obliged to cooperate closely in abortions and have to choose between the law of God and their professional situation.

—Congregation for the Doctrine of the Faith,
Declaration on Procured Abortion, 22

28. Does the Church tell us what should be done for those tempted by abortion?

It is the task of law to pursue a reform of society and of conditions of life in all milieux, starting with the most deprived, so that always and everywhere it may be possible to give every child coming into this world a welcome worthy of a person. Help for families and for unmarried mothers, assured grants for children, a statute for illegitimate children and reasonable arrangements for adoption—a whole positive policy must be put into force so that there will always be a concrete, honorable, and possible alternative to abortion.

—Congregation for the Doctrine of the Faith,
Declaration on Procured Abortion, 23

29. Would not the availability of contraception mean a reduction in abortions? Why then does the Church not allow for contraceptive use at least to avoid abortion?

EDITOR'S NOTE: The issue of preventing fertility is further addressed below. This question pertains to a claim that surfaces in discussion on abortion. ✣

Contraception uses all the means at its disposal to prevent a new life from coming into existence. If, despite the contraception, a new life is engendered, it is often rejected and aborted. Contraception, far from making abortion less common, finds therein its logical extension.

—Pontifical Council for Pastoral Assistance to Health Care Workers,
New Charter for Health Care Workers, 19

It is frequently asserted that *contraception*, if made safe and available to all, is the most effective remedy against abortion. . . . When looked at carefully, this objection is clearly unfounded. It may be that many people use contraception with a view to exclude the subsequent temptation of abortion. But the negative values inherent in the "contraceptive mentality"—which is very different from responsible parenthood, lived in respect for the full truth of the conjugal act—are such that they in fact strengthen this temptation when an unwanted life is conceived. Indeed, the pro-abortion culture is especially strong precisely where the Church's teaching on contraception is rejected. Certainly, from the moral point of view contraception and abortion are *specifically different* evils: the former contradicts the full truth of the sexual act as the proper expression of conjugal love, while the latter destroys the life of a human being; the former is opposed to the virtue of chastity in marriage, the latter is opposed to the virtue of justice and directly violates the divine commandment "You shall not kill."

But despite their differences of nature and moral gravity, contraception and abortion are often closely connected, as fruits of the same tree. It is true that in many cases contraception and even abortion are practiced under the pressure of real-life difficulties, which nonetheless can never exonerate from striving to observe God's law fully. Still, in very many other instances such practices are rooted in a hedonistic mentality unwilling to accept responsibility in matters of sexuality, and they imply a self-centered concept of freedom, which regards procreation as an obstacle to personal fulfillment. The life which could result from a sexual encounter thus becomes an enemy to be avoided at all costs, and abortion becomes the only possible decisive response to failed contraception.

—John Paul II, *Evangelium vitae*, 13

30. What if ending a pregnancy is needed to save the life of the mother such as is the case with an ectopic pregnancy?

EDITOR'S NOTE: An ectopic pregnancy is one in which the developing child implants outside of the uterine cavity. If she or he continues to develop, this can cause a rupture (e.g., in the fallopian tube) which can cause life threatening hemorrhaging. ✢

Any form of direct abortion is ethically illegitimate inasmuch as it is an intrinsically reprehensible act. When abortion is neither intended nor willed but follows as a foreseen consequence of a therapeutic act that is inescapably necessary for the health of the mother, this may be morally legitimate. In such a case, the abortion is the indirect consequence of an act that in itself is not a direct abortion.

—Pontifical Council for Pastoral Assistance to Health Care Workers,
New Charter for Health Care Workers, 54

Here [in the case of ectopic pregnancy] the applicable norm prohibits interventions to directly destroy the embryo, while it justifies interventions aimed exclusively at preserving the life and health of the woman that result in the embryo's demise.

—Pontifical Council for Pastoral Assistance to Health Care Workers,
New Charter for Health Care Workers, 57

Operations, treatments, and medications that have as their direct purpose the cure of a proportionately serious pathological condition of a pregnant woman are permitted when they cannot be safely postponed until the unborn child is viable, even if they will result in the death of the unborn child.

In case of extrauterine pregnancy, no intervention is morally licit which constitutes a direct abortion.

For a proportionate reason, labor may be induced after the fetus is viable.

—USCCB, *Ethical and Religious Directives
for Catholic Health Care Services*, 47–49

31. Is it permissible to cooperate in a direct abortion such as providing pre-operation nursing care, or anesthesia?

EDITOR'S NOTE: What is said in answers to questions 31–33 pertain specifically to Catholic hospitals situated within a broader secular healthcare delivery system. What is said in these quotations is analogous to what can be said about a Catholic clinician working within an institution that permits immoral procedures. Both can be understood as "agents," the root etymology of which comes from the Latin *agens* meaning "to act." And both are acting within a web of other agents. The same principles of cooperation apply whether the agent is corporate or individual. Issues of scandal, however, might require a different analysis between individuals and corporations because of the greater public visibility of the latter. ✢

Medical and healthcare integrity declares illegitimate any surgical or pharmaceutical intervention aimed at interrupting pregnancy at any stage.

—Pontifical Council for Pastoral Assistance to Health Care Workers,
New Charter for Health Care Workers, 52

Catholic healthcare institutions are not to provide abortion services, even based upon the principle of material cooperation.

—USCCB, *Ethical and Religious Directives
for Catholic Health Care Services*, 45

EDITOR'S NOTE: Material cooperation means the assistance in the evil act of another but without the intention for the evil act. It is called "material" because one is providing the "matter" or ingredients that facilitate an evil act, such as providing anesthesia services for a direct sterilization, or nursing preoperatory care for a direct abortion. Neither preoperatory care nor anesthesia are themselves an act of direct abortion, but they are causally related to it. ✢

Catholic healthcare organizations are not permitted to engage in immediate material cooperation in actions that are intrinsically immoral, such as abortion, euthanasia, assisted suicide, and direct sterilization.

—USCCB, *Ethical and Religious Directives
for Catholic Health Care Services*, 70

The opportunity to refuse to take part [in direct abortions and euthanasia] in the phases of consultation, preparation, and execution of these acts against life should be guaranteed to physicians, healthcare personnel, and directors of hospitals, clinics, and convalescent facilities.

—John Paul II, *Evangelium vitae*, 74

32. Can a Catholic doctor work at an institution that performs abortions? Is he or she obliged to try to find another job?

A Catholic hospital contemplating joining a healthcare system that permits immoral procedures must, before entering into any such agreement, ensure that neither its administrators nor its employees will be involved directly in immoral procedures undertaken by other institutions within the system. It must also ensure that its facilities and other resources will not be utilized in such procedures and that no administrator or employee will be obliged to make referrals for immoral procedures. Great care must be exercised to avoid giving scandal.

—Congregation for the Doctrine of the Faith,
"Principles for Collaboration with Non-Catholic Entities," 9

33. If a Catholic doctor is ordered to participate in a procedure against Church teaching, under penalty of losing his or her employment, what should he or she do?

A human being can never obey an intrinsically immoral law, as is the case with a law that admitted, as a matter of principle, that abortion is licit. The force of the inviolability of human life and of God's law, which defends it, precedes any positive human law.

—Pontifical Council for Pastoral Assistance to Health Care Workers,
New Charter for Health Care Workers, 59

To refuse to take part in committing an injustice is not only a moral duty; it is also a basic human right. Were this not so, the human person would be forced to perform an action intrinsically incompatible with human dignity, and in this way human freedom itself, the authentic meaning and purpose of which are found in its orientation to the true and the good, would be radically compromised.

—John Paul II, *Evangelium vitae*, 74

Besides being a sign of professional integrity, a healthcare worker's earnestly motivated conscientious objection has the noble significance of *a social denunciation of a legal injustice* that is being perpetrated against innocent and defenseless lives.

—Pontifical Council for Pastoral Assistance to Health Care Workers, *New Charter for Health Care Workers*, 60

Conceived in Love

34. What ethical values guide decision making on treating infertility?

The fundamental values connected with the techniques of artificial human procreation are two: the life of the human being called into existence and the special nature of the transmission of human life in marriage.

—Congregation for the Doctrine of the Faith, *Donum vitae*, introduction, 4

With regard to the *treatment of infertility*, new medical techniques must respect three fundamental goods: a) the right to life and to physical integrity of every human being from conception to natural death; b) the unity of marriage, which means reciprocal respect for the right within marriage to become a father or mother only together with the other spouse; c) the specifically human values of sexuality which require "that the procreation of a human person be brought about as the fruit of the conjugal act specific to the love between spouses."

—Congregation for the Doctrine of the Faith, *Dignitas personae*, 12 (quoting Congregation for the Doctrine of the Faith, *Donum vitae*, II.4)

Human procreation has specific characteristics by virtue of the personal dignity of the parents and of the children: the procreation of a new person, whereby the man and the woman collaborate with the power of the Creator, must be the fruit and the sign of the mutual self-giving of the spouses, of their love, and of their fidelity.

—Congregation for the Doctrine of the Faith, *Donum vitae*, II.1

Respect for the unity of marriage and for conjugal fidelity demands that the child be conceived in marriage; the bond existing between husband and wife accords the spouses, in an objective and inalienable manner, the exclusive right to become father and mother solely through each other.

—Congregation for the Doctrine of the Faith, *Donum vitae*, II.2

From the moral point of view procreation is deprived of its proper perfection when it is not desired as the fruit of the conjugal act, that is to say of the specific act of the spouses' union.

—Congregation for the Doctrine of the Faith, *Donum vitae*, II.4.a

The moral relevance of the link between the meanings of the conjugal act and between the goods of marriage, as well as the unity of the human being and the dignity of his origin, demand that the procreation of a human person be brought about as the fruit of the conjugal act specific to the love between spouses.

—Congregation for the Doctrine of the Faith, *Donum vitae*, II.4.c

When the marital act of sexual intercourse is not able to attain its procreative purpose, assistance that does not separate the unitive and procreative ends of the act, and does not substitute for the marital act itself, may be used to help married couples conceive.

—USCCB, *Ethical and Religious Directives for Catholic Health Care Services*, 38

The moral criteria for medical intervention in procreation are deduced from the dignity of human persons, of their sexuality and of their origin. *Medicine which seeks to be ordered to the integral good of the person must respect the specifically human values of sexuality. The doctor is at the service of persons and of human procreation. He does not have the authority to dispose of them or to decide their fate.*

—Congregation for the Doctrine of the faith, *Donum vitae*, II.7

35. How should the good of the "unity of marriage" be understood?

The fidelity of the spouses in the unity of marriage involves reciprocal respect of their right to become a father and a mother only through each other. The child has the right to be conceived, carried in the womb, brought into the world and brought up within marriage: it is through the secure and recognized relationship to his own parents that the child can discover his own identity and achieve his own proper human development. The parents find in their child a confirmation and completion of their reciprocal self-giving: the child is the living image of their love, the permanent sign of their conjugal union, the living and indissoluble concrete expression of their paternity and maternity.

—Congregation for the Doctrine of the Faith, *Donum vitae*, II.1

Marriage and conjugal love are by their nature ordained toward the begetting and educating of children.

—Vatican Council II, *Gaudium et spes*, 50

The intimate partnership of married life and love has been established by the Creator and qualified by His laws, and is rooted in the conjugal covenant of irrevocable personal consent. Hence by that human act whereby spouses mutually bestow and accept each other a relationship arises which by divine will and in the eyes of society too is a lasting one. For the good of the spouses and their offspring as well as of society, the existence of the sacred bond no longer depends on human decisions alone. For, God Himself is the author of matrimony, endowed as it is with various benefits and purposes. All of these have a very decisive bearing on the continuation of the human race, on the personal development and eternal destiny of the individual members of a family, and on the dignity, stability, peace, and prosperity of the family itself and of human society as a whole. By their very nature, the institution of matrimony itself and conjugal love are ordained for the procreation and education of children, and find in them their ultimate crown.

—Vatican Council II, *Gaudium et spes*, 48

36. How should the good of "procreation" and its essential connection to conjugal union be understood?

In the biblical narrative, the difference between man and other creatures is shown above all by the fact that only the creation of man is presented as the result of a special decision on the part of God, a deliberation to establish *a particular and specific bond with the Creator*: "Let us make man in our image, after our likeness" (Gen 1:26). *The life* which God offers to man *is a gift by which God shares something of himself with his creature.*

—John Paul II, *Evangelium vitae*, 34

The fundamental task of the family is to serve life, to actualize in history the original blessing of the Creator—that of transmitting by procreation the divine image from person to person.

—John Paul II, *Familiaris consortio*, 28

In affirming that the spouses, as parents, cooperate with God the Creator in conceiving and giving birth to a new human being, we are not speaking merely with reference to the laws of biology.... Begetting is the continuation of Creation.

—John Paul II, *Evangelium vitae*, 43

Human procreation has specific characteristics by virtue of the personal dignity of the parents and of the children: the procreation of a new person, whereby the man and the woman collaborate with the power of the Creator, must be the fruit and the sign of the mutual self-giving of the spouses, of their love and of their fidelity. The fidelity of the spouses in the unity of marriage involves reciprocal respect of their right to become a father and a mother only through each other. The child has the right to be conceived, carried in the womb, brought into the world, and brought up within marriage: it is through the secure and recognized relationship to his own parents that the child can discover his own identity and achieve his own proper human development.... By reason of the vocation and social responsibilities of the person, the good of the children and of the parents contributes to the good of civil society; the vitality and stability of society require that children come into the world within a family and that the family be firmly based on marriage. The tradition of the Church and anthropological reflection recognize in marriage and in its indissoluble unity the only setting worthy of truly responsible procreation.

—Congregation for the Doctrine of the Faith, *Donum vitae*, II.1

The Church's teaching on marriage and human procreation affirms the "inseparable connection, willed by God and unable to be broken by man on his own initiative, between the two meanings of the conjugal act: the unitive meaning and the procreative meaning. Indeed, by its intimate structure, the conjugal act, while most closely uniting husband

and wife, capacitates them for the generation of new lives, according to laws inscribed in the very being of man and of woman."

> —Congregation for the Doctrine of the Faith, *Donum vitae*, II.4.a
> (quoting Paul VI, *Humanae vitae*, 12)

The moral value of the intimate link between the goods of marriage and between the meanings of the conjugal act is based upon the unity of the human being, a unity involving body and spiritual soul. . . . It is an act that is inseparably corporal and spiritual. It is in their bodies and through their bodies that the spouses consummate their marriage and are able to become father and mother.

> —Congregation for the Doctrine of the Faith, *Donum vitae*, II.4.b

Only respect for the link between the meanings of the conjugal act and respect for the unity of the human being make possible procreation in conformity with the dignity of the person. In his unique and irrepeatable origin, the child must be respected and recognized as equal in personal dignity to those who give him life. The human person must be accepted in his parents' act of union and love; the generation of a child must therefore be the fruit of that mutual giving.

> —Congregation for the Doctrine of the Faith, *Donum vitae*, II.4.c

Conception and Infertility

EDITOR'S NOTE: For the purposes of the following set of questions several terms and procedures require explanation. Treatments for infertility are divided into two categories: artificial and natural. "Natural means" does not entail only non-medical means, but rather, it refers to those means that *assist in* but do not *replace* the conjugal act. Surgical correction for a blocked fallopian tube, for example, is natural in this sense. Artificial means are those that replace the capacity of the conjugal act. In vitro fertilization (IVF) is a common artificial means since conception takes place apart from any specific conjugal union of the spouses. (In vitro means "in the glass"). The Church also distinguishes between homologous IVF (using the sperm and oocytes from each spouse joined in marriage) and heterologous IVF (using sperm or oocyte from a person not joined in marriage to one of the spouses). The Church has offered ethical commentary on the following four principal stages of IVF procedures, and the organization below follows the same pattern.

The *first stage* of IVF procedures is the *collection* of gametes. This typically involves collecting male gametes by masturbation, aspirating oocytes from the woman, usually several, with the goal of having several human beings conceived in vitro—referred to as "embryos" as if they are some different kind of thing than you and me. It is more accurate to understand them as human beings at the embryonic stage of development. The *second stage* is *conception in vitro*. The *third stage* is the *selection* of embryos. This includes performing, though not in all cases, pre-implantation genetic diagnosis to select the child for hair color, propensity for genetic diseases, etc. It also includes selecting one or more embryos for transfer to the mother's uterus for possible implantation. The *fourth stage* is the *disposition* of embryos. Often, several embryos are not chosen for implantation and are pejoratively called "left over" or "spare" embryos. They are either frozen, often interminably; destroyed; or destroyed for research purposes. Sometimes couples elect to have more than one or two human beings transferred to increase the likelihood of implantation. If all implant, it is common to perform a practice called "selective reduction" or "embryo reduction" which is an act of directly killing one or more of the implanted children, usually between 9 and 12 weeks gestation. The Church provides ethical commentary on each stage and their principal aspects. ✢

Certainly, techniques aimed at removing obstacles to natural fertilization, as for example, hormonal treatments for infertility, surgery for endometriosis, unblocking of fallopian tubes or their surgical repair, are licit. All these techniques may be considered *authentic treatments* because, once the problem causing the infertility has been resolved, the married couple is able to engage in conjugal acts resulting in procreation, without the physician's action directly interfering in that act itself. None of these treatments replaces the conjugal act, which alone is worthy of truly responsible procreation.

—Congregation for the Doctrine of the Faith, *Dignitas personae*, 13

37. Is the way in which gametes are collected for the purposes of creating new human life permissible?

Masturbation is an intrinsically and seriously disordered act. The main reason is that, whatever the motive for acting this way, the deliberate use of the sexual faculty outside normal conjugal relations essentially contradicts the finality of the faculty. For it lacks the sexual relationship called for by the moral order, namely the relationship which realizes "the full sense of mutual self-giving and human procreation in the context of true love."

—Congregation for the Doctrine of the Faith, *Persona humana*, 9
(quoting Vatican Council II, *Gaudium et spes*, 51)

Artificial insemination as a substitute for the conjugal act is prohibited by reason of the voluntarily achieved dissociation of the two meanings of the conjugal act. Masturbation, through which the sperm is normally obtained, is another sign of this dissociation: even when it is done for the purpose of procreation, the act remains deprived of its unitive meaning.

—Congregation for the Doctrine of the Faith, *Donum vitae*, II.6

38. Is the second stage of conception via in vitro fertilization using heterologous gametes permissible?

Heterologous artificial fertilization is contrary to the unity of marriage, to the dignity of the spouses, to the vocation proper to parents, and to the child's right to be conceived and brought into the world in marriage and from marriage.... Consequently fertilization of a married woman with the sperm of a donor different from her husband and fertilization with the husband's sperm of an ovum not coming from his wife are morally illicit. Furthermore, the artificial fertilization of a woman who is unmarried or a widow, whoever the donor may be, cannot be morally justified.

—Congregation for the Doctrine of the Faith, *Donum vitae*, II.2

39. Is the second stage of conception in vitro using homologous gametes permissible?

Conception *in vitro* is the result of the technical action which presides over fertilization. *Such fertilization is neither in fact achieved nor positively willed as the expression and fruit of a specific act of the conjugal union. In homologous IVF and ET [embryo transfer], therefore, even if it is considered in the context of "de facto" existing sexual relations, the generation of the human person is objectively deprived of its proper perfection: namely, that of being the result and fruit of a conjugal act in* which the spouses can become "cooperators with God for giving life to a new person."

—Congregation for the Doctrine of the Faith, *Donum vitae*, II.5 (quoting John Paul II, *Familiaris consortio*, 14)

Techniques of fertilization *in vitro* can open the way to other forms of biological and genetic manipulation of human embryos , ... *These procedures are contrary to the human dignity proper to the embryo, and at the same time they are contrary to the right of every person to be conceived and to be born within marriage and from marriage.*

—Congregation for the Doctrine of the Faith, *Donum vitae*, I.6

No one, before coming into existence, can claim a subjective right to begin to exist; nevertheless, it is legitimate to affirm the right of the child to have a fully human origin through conception in conformity with the personal nature of the human being. Life is a gift that must be bestowed in a manner worthy both of the subject receiving it and of the subjects transmitting it.

—Congregation for the Doctrine of the Faith, *Donum vitae*, I.6n32

In reality, the origin of a human person is the result of an act of giving. The one conceived must be the fruit of his parents' love. He cannot be desired or conceived as the product of an intervention of medical or biological techniques; that would be equivalent to reducing him to an object of scientific technology. No one may subject the coming of a child into the world to conditions of technical efficiency which are to be evaluated according to standards of control and dominion.

—Congregation for the Doctrine of the Faith, *Donum vitae*, II.4.c

40. Is the third stage of selecting embryos for transfer permissible?

The reason for multiple transfer is to increase the probability that at least one embryo will implant in the uterus. In this technique, therefore, the number of embryos transferred is greater than the single child desired, in the expectation that some embryos will be lost and multiple pregnancy may not occur. In this way, the practice of multiple embryo transfer implies *a purely utilitarian treatment of embryos....*

This sad reality, which often goes unmentioned, is truly deplorable: the "various techniques of artificial reproduction, which would seem to be at the service of life and which are frequently used with this intention, actually open the door to new threats against life."

—Congregation for the Doctrine of the Faith, *Dignitas personae*, 15
(quoting John Paul II, *Evangelium vitae*, 14)

Embryonic Human Beings

41. Is pre-implantation diagnosis permissible?

Preimplantation diagnosis—connected as it is with artificial fertilization, which is itself always intrinsically illicit—is directed toward the *qualitative selection and consequent destruction of embryos*, which constitutes an act of abortion. Preimplantation diagnosis is therefore the expression of a *eugenic mentality* that "accepts selective abortion in order to prevent the birth of children affected by various types of anomalies. Such an attitude is shameful and utterly reprehensible, since it presumes to measure the value of a human life only within the parameters of 'normality' and physical well-being, thus opening the way to legitimizing infanticide and euthanasia as well."

—Congregation for the Doctrine of the Faith, *Dignitas personae*, 22
(quoting John Paul II, *Evangelium vitae*, 63)

42. Is freezing embryos in the fourth stage permissible?

Cryopreservation is *incompatible with the respect owed to human embryos*; it presupposes their production *in vitro*; it exposes them to the serious risk of death or physical harm, since a high percentage does not survive the process of freezing and thawing; it deprives them at least temporarily of maternal reception and gestation; it places them in a situation in which they are susceptible to further offense and manipulation.

—Congregation for the Doctrine of the Faith, *Dignitas personae*, 18

43. Is the disposition phase permissible when the embryo is destroyed, or destroyed for research purposes?

It is true that approximately a third of women who have recourse to artificial procreation succeed in having a baby. It should be recognized, however, that given the proportion between the total number of embryos produced and those eventually born, *the number of embryos sacrificed is extremely high* [about 80%]. These losses are accepted by the practitioners of in vitro fertilization as the price to be paid for positive results. In reality, it is deeply disturbing that research in this area aims principally at obtaining better results in terms of the percentage of babies born to women who begin the process, but does not manifest a concrete interest in the right to life of each individual embryo.

—Congregation for the Doctrine of the Faith, *Dignitas personae*, 14

These techniques [i.e., IVF] in fact involve *the loss of many embryos.* Some of these losses result from the techniques themselves, whereby the loss of around 80 percent of the embryos that are actually transferred is accepted in order to obtain the birth of one baby. Other embryos are eliminated directly because they have genetic defects. Finally, in the case of a multiple pregnancy, one or more embryos or fetuses may be destroyed directly to reduce risks to the embryos or fetuses that are spared. Every direct destruction of a human being between conception and birth has the character of an actual abortion in the moral sense.

—Pontifical Council for Pastoral Assistance to Health Care Workers, *New Charter for Health Care Workers*, 28

The dignity of a person must be recognized in every human being from conception to natural death. This fundamental principle expresses *a great "yes" to human life* and must be at the center of ethical reflection on biomedical research, which has an ever greater importance in today's world.

—Congregation for the Doctrine of the Faith, *Dignitas personae*, 1

The human being must be respected—as a person—from the very first instant of his existence....
The fruit of human generation, from the first moment of its existence, that is to say from the moment the zygote has formed, demands the unconditional respect that is morally due to the human being in his bodily and spiritual totality. The human being is to be respected and treated as a person from the moment of conception; and therefore from that same moment his rights as a person must be recognized, among which in the first place is the inviolable right of every innocent human being to life.

—Congregation for the Doctrine of the Faith, *Donum vitae*, I.1

In the circumstances in which it is regularly practiced, IVF and ET involves the destruction of human beings, which is something contrary to the doctrine on the illicitness of abortion.

—Congregation for the Doctrine of the Faith, *Donum vitae*, II.5

44. Is IVF permissible if care is taken to ensure that all human beings conceived are transferred in hopes that all implant, gestate, and are born?

The so-called simple case, i.e., a homologous IVF and ET procedure that is free of any compromise with the abortive practice of destroying embryos and with masturbation, remains a technique which is morally illicit because it deprives human procreation of the dignity which is proper and connatural to it.

—Congregation for the Doctrine of the Faith *Donum vitae*, II.5

Even in a situation in which every precaution were taken to avoid the death of human embryos, homologous IVF and ET dissociate from the conjugal act the actions which are directed to human fertilization . . . . *The Church remains opposed from the moral point of view to homologous "in vitro" fertilization. Such fertilization is in itself illicit and in opposition to the dignity of procreation and of the conjugal union, even when everything is done to avoid the death of the human embryo.*

—Congregation for the Doctrine of the Faith, *Donum vitae*, II.5

45. Is selective/embryo reduction permissible?

From the ethical point of view, *embryo reduction is an intentional selective abortion.* It is in fact the deliberate and direct elimination of one or more innocent human beings in the initial phase of their existence and as such it always constitutes a grave moral disorder.

The ethical justifications proposed for embryo reduction are often based on analogies with natural disasters or emergency situations in which, despite the best intentions of all involved, it is not possible to save everyone. Such analogies cannot in any way be the basis for an action which is directly abortive. At other times, moral principles are invoked, such as those of the lesser evil or double effect, which are likewise inapplicable in this case. It is never permitted to do something which is intrinsically illicit, not even in view of a good result: *the end does not justify the means.*

—Congregation for the Doctrine of the Faith, *Dignitas personae*, 21

46. In light of roughly 500,000 "spare" embryos currently cryogenically frozen, is embryo or "prenatal" adoption permissible?

With regard to the large number of *frozen embryos already in existence* the question becomes: what to do with them?...

The proposal that these embryos could be put at the disposal of infertile couples as a *treatment for infertility* is not ethically acceptable for the same reasons which make artificial heterologous procreation illicit as well as any form of surrogate motherhood; this practice would also lead to other problems of a medical, psychological, and legal nature.

It has also been proposed, solely in order to allow human beings to be born who are otherwise condemned to destruction, that there could be a form of "prenatal adoption." This proposal, praiseworthy with regard to the intention of respecting and defending human life, presents however various problems not dissimilar to those mentioned above. All things considered, it needs to be recognized that the thousands of abandoned embryos represent a *situation of injustice which in fact cannot be resolved.*

—Congregation for the Doctrine of the Faith, *Dignitas personae*, 19

47. Is the Church against all forms of reproductive technology?

In light of this principle, all techniques of heterologous artificial fertilization, as well as those techniques of homologous artificial fertilization which substitute for the conjugal act, are to be excluded. On the other hand, techniques which act *as an aid to the conjugal act and its fertility* are permitted.

—Congregation for the Doctrine of the Faith, *Dignitas personae*, 12

Certainly, techniques aimed at removing obstacles to natural fertilization, as for example, hormonal treatments for infertility, surgery for endometriosis, unblocking of fallopian tubes or their surgical repair, are licit. All these techniques may be considered *authentic treatments* because, once the problem causing the infertility has been resolved, the married couple is able to engage in conjugal acts resulting in procreation, without the physician's action directly interfering in that act itself. None of these treatments replaces the conjugal act, which alone is worthy of truly responsible procreation.

—Congregation for the Doctrine of the Faith, *Dignitas personae*, 13

48. Is sperm and egg donation morally permitted as in cases involving surrogate motherhood or even insemination by a deceased husband's sperm?

Surrogate motherhood is equally contrary to the dignity of the woman, to the unity of marriage, and to the dignity of the procreation of a human person.

To impregnate a woman by fertilizing her own ovum with donor sperm or by implanting into a woman's uterus an embryo that is genetically foreign to her, and to make her promise to deliver the newborn child to a client, is to fragment motherhood, reducing gestation to a process of incubation that shows no respect for the child's dignity and "right to be conceived, carried in the womb, brought into the world, and brought up within marriage."

—Pontifical Council for Pastoral Assistance to Health Care Workers, *New Charter for Health Care Workers*, 31 (quoting Congregation for the Doctrine of the Faith, *Donum vitae*, II.1)

49. Is it permissible to engage in reproductive cloning?

EDITOR'S NOTE: Human cloning involves removing the nucleus of an oocyte (egg cell) and replacing it with the nucleus of a living person's somatic (body or skin) cell. The resulting oocyte is then cultured and stimulated in a way that is meant to mimic fertilization and trigger normal human development. Reproductive cloning transfers the human being to a uterus in order to implant, gestate, and be born. Therapeutic cloning destroys the cloned human being to harvest genetically matched organs or tissues for the person whose cells were used for cloning. ✛

Human cloning is intrinsically illicit in that, by taking the ethical negativity of techniques of artificial fertilization to their extreme, it seeks to *give rise to a new human being without a connection to the act of reciprocal self-giving between the spouses* and, more radically, *without any link to sexuality.*

—Congregation for the Doctrine of the Faith, *Dignitas personae*, 28

Suffering Infertility

50. Is not the will or desire for a child a good one? So, if care is taken to bring into being through IVF only one embryo and transfer him or her to the mother, is that still wrong?

The desire for a child does not give rise to any right to a child. A child is a person, with the dignity of a "subject." As such he cannot be willed as an "object" of a right. Rather, the child is the subject of rights: it is the child's right to be conceived with full respect for the fact that he is a person.

—Pontifical Council for Pastoral Assistance to Health Care Workers,
New Charter for Health Care Workers, 27

A child is not something owed to one but is a *gift*. The "supreme gift of marriage" is a human person. A child may not be considered a piece of property, an idea to which an alleged "right to a child" would lead. In this area, only the child possesses genuine rights: the right "to be the fruit of the specific act of the conjugal love of his parents," and "the right to be respected as a person from the moment of his conception."

—*Catechism of the Catholic Church*, 2378
(quoting Congregation for the Doctrine of the Faith, *Donum vitae*, II.8)

51. What pastoral guidance can be given couples who suffer infertility?

Whatever its cause or prognosis, sterility is certainly a difficult trial. The community of believers is called to shed light upon and support the suffering of those who are unable to fulfill their legitimate aspiration to motherhood and fatherhood. Spouses who find themselves in this sad situation are called to find in it an opportunity for sharing in a particular way in the Lord's Cross, the source of spiritual fruitfulness. Sterile couples must not forget that "even when procreation is not possible, conjugal life does not for this reason lose its value. Physical sterility in fact can be for spouses the occasion for other important services to the life of the human person, for example, adoption, various forms of educational work, and assistance to other families and to poor or handicapped children."

—Congregation for the Doctrine of the Faith, *Donum vitae*, II.8
(quoting John Paul II, *Familiaris consortio*, 14)

Loving One's Spouse

52. What values should be respected when thinking about the regulation of one's fertility?

[Deciding to have or not to have more children] gives rise to the need for a way of regulating fertility that is an expression of conscious and responsible openness to the transmission of life.

In evaluating actions with regard to this regulation, ... this is a question of the dignity of the man and the woman and of their intimate relationship. Respect for this dignity characterizes the truth of conjugal love.

—Pontifical Council for Pastoral Assistance to Health Care Workers,
New Charter for Health Care Workers, 14–15

The true practice of conjugal love, and the whole meaning of the family life which results from it, have this aim: that the couple be ready with stout hearts to cooperate with the love of the Creator and the Savior, who through them will enlarge and enrich His own family day by day.

—Vatican Council II, *Gaudium et spes*, 50

Married love particularly reveals its true nature and nobility when we realize that it takes its origin from God, who "is love." ... As a consequence, husband and wife, through that mutual gift of themselves, which is specific and exclusive to them alone, develop that union of two persons in which they perfect one another, cooperating with God in the generation and rearing of new lives.

—Paul VI, *Humanae vitae*, 8

With regard to the biological processes, responsible parenthood means an awareness of, and respect for, their proper functions. In the procreative faculty the human mind discerns biological laws that apply to the human person.

With regard to man's innate drives and emotions, responsible parenthood means that man's reason and will must exert control over them.

With regard to physical, economic, psychological, and social conditions, responsible parenthood is exercised by those who prudently and generously decide to have more children, and by those who, for serious reasons and with due respect to moral precepts, decide not to have additional children for either a certain or an indefinite period of time.

—Paul VI, *Humanae vitae*, 10

The Church, nevertheless, in urging men to the observance of the precepts of the natural law, which it interprets by its constant doctrine, teaches that each and every marital act must of necessity retain its intrinsic relationship to the procreation of human life.

This particular doctrine, ... is based on the inseparable connection, ... between the unitive significance and the procreative significance which are both inherent to the marriage act. The reason is that the fundamental nature of the marriage act, while uniting husband and wife in the closest intimacy, also renders them capable of generating new life—and this as a result of laws written into the actual nature of man and of woman. And if each of these essential qualities, the unitive and the procreative, is preserved, the use of marriage fully retains its sense of true mutual love and its ordination to the supreme responsibility of parenthood to which man is called.

—Paul VI, *Humanae vitae*, 11–12

53. Is the direct (or intentional) use of artificial means for preventing fertilization permissible?

Direct sterilization of either men or women, whether permanent [e.g., tubal ligation] or temporary [e.g., oral contraceptive pills], is not permitted in a Catholic healthcare institution.

—USCCB, *Ethical and Religious Directives for Catholic Health Care Services*, 53

Any sterilization which of itself, that is, of its own nature and condition, has the sole immediate effect of rendering the generative faculty incapable of procreation, is to be considered a direct sterilization. ... Such sterilization remains absolutely forbidden according to the doctrine of the Church.

—Congregation for the Doctrine of the Faith, *Quaecumque sterilizatio*, 1

Equally to be condemned, as the magisterium of the Church has affirmed on many occasions, is direct sterilization, whether of the man or of the woman, whether permanent or temporary.

Similarly excluded is any action which either before, at the moment of, or after sexual intercourse, is specifically intended to prevent procreation—whether as an end or as a means.

—Paul VI, *Humanae vitae*, 14

No reason, however grave, may be put forward by which anything intrinsically against nature may become conformable to nature and morally good. Since, therefore, the conjugal act is destined primarily by nature for the begetting of children, those who in exercising it deliberately frustrate its natural power and purpose sin against nature and commit a deed which is shameful and intrinsically vicious.

—Pius XI, *Casti connubii*, 54

Any use whatsoever of matrimony exercised in such a way that the act is deliberately frustrated in its natural power to generate life is an offense against the law of God and of nature, and those who indulge in such are branded with the guilt of a grave sin.

—Pius XI, *Casti connubii*, 56

The acts themselves which are proper to conjugal love and which are exercised in accord with genuine human dignity must be honored with great reverence. Hence when there is question of harmonizing conjugal love with the responsible transmission of life, the moral aspects of any procedure does not depend solely on sincere intentions or on an evaluation of motives, but must be determined by objective standards. These, based on the nature of the human person and his acts, preserve the full sense of mutual self-giving and human procreation in the context of true love. Such a goal cannot be achieved unless the virtue of conjugal chastity is sincerely practiced. Relying on these principles, sons of the Church may not undertake methods of birth control which are found blameworthy by the teaching authority of the Church in its unfolding of the divine law.

—Vatican Council II, *Gaudium et spes*, 51

The precise object of sterilization is to impede the functioning of the reproductive organs, and the malice of sterilization consists in the refusal of children: it is an act against the *bonum prolis* [i.e., the good of progeny or children].

—Congregation for the Doctrine of the Faith,
Response to a Question on the Liceity of a Hysterectomy in Certain Cases

Prescriptions and Medical Procedures

54. Why would the Church say it is immoral for a physician to prescribe oral contraceptive drugs or other contraceptive products? Shouldn't that be the patient's decision?

EDITOR'S NOTE: This question is not about the morality of using contraceptives—see the previous question—but about the physician's action of *prescribing* them for contraceptive purposes. ✢

Catholic healthcare organizations are not permitted to engage in immediate material cooperation in actions that are intrinsically immoral, such as abortion, euthanasia, assisted suicide, and direct sterilization.

—USCCB, *Ethical and Religious Directives
for Catholic Health Care Services*, 70

EDITOR'S NOTE: Ethical teaching that is explicitly about Catholic organizations also applies to individuals—the only possible exceptions being issues of scandal due to the public visibility of organizations. An individual who performs an objectively permissible act which could be misinterpreted does not act scandalously if the act is not "visible" to others. ✢

55. When a drug is prescribed for the treatment of a condition or disease and it is associated with a risk for birth defects, is it permissible to prescribe contraceptives also?

Direct sterilization of either men or women, whether permanent [e.g., tubal ligation] or temporary [e.g., contraceptive pills], is not permitted in a Catholic healthcare institution. Procedures that induce sterility are permitted when their direct effect is the cure or alleviation of a present and serious pathology and a simpler treatment is not available.

—USCCB, *Ethical and Religious Directives
for Catholic Health Care Services*, 53

56. Is the use of oral contraceptive pills permissible in cases of rape?

Compassionate and understanding care should be given to a person who is the victim of sexual assault. Healthcare providers should cooperate with law enforcement officials and offer the person psychological and spiritual support as well as accurate medical information. A female who has been raped should be able to defend herself against a potential conception from the sexual assault. If, after appropriate testing, there is no evidence that conception has occurred already, she may be treated with medications that would prevent ovulation, sperm capacitation, or fertilization. It is not permissible, however, to initiate or to recommend treatments that have as their purpose or direct effect the removal, destruction, or interference with the implantation of a fertilized ovum.

—USCCB, *Ethical and Religious Directives for Catholic Health Care Services*, 36

57. Is the use of sterilizing measures, either permanent or temporary, permissible for those who have mental disability or mental illness?

Notwithstanding any subjectively right intention of those whose actions are prompted by the care or prevention of physical or mental illness which is foreseen or feared as a result of pregnancy, such sterilization remains absolutely forbidden according to the doctrine of the Church.

—Congregation for the Doctrine of the Faith, *Quaecumque sterilizatio*, 1

58. Is the use of contraceptive methods permissible to prevent the conception of a child who will likely inherit a genetically inheritable disease from one of the parents?

Several times already We have taken a position on the subject of sterilization. We have stated, in substance, that direct sterilization is not authorized by man's right to dispose of his own body and therefore cannot be considered as a valid way to prevent transmission of a hereditary disease. "Direct sterilization," We said on October 29, 1951 [address to midwives], . . . "which aims, as a means or as an end, at rendering procreation impossible, is a grave violation of the moral law, and is therefore illicit."

—Pius XII, "Morality and Eugenics," Address to the Participants in the Seventh Congress of the International Society of Hematology, September 12, 1958

59. Is it permissible to use contraceptive pills to remedy excessive uterine spasms (menstrual cramps)?

If a woman takes such medicine, not to prevent conception, but only on the advice of the doctor, as a necessary remedy because of the condition of the uterus or the organism, she produces *indirect* sterilization, which is permitted according to the general principles governing acts with a double effect.

—Pius XII, "Morality and Eugenics," Address to the participants in the seventh Congress of the International Society of Hematology, September 12, 1958

60. Is it permissible to use contraceptive pills to prevent pregnancy because it is known that the uterus would not be able to bear a developing human being?

A *direct* and, therefore, illicit sterilization results when ovulation is stopped to protect the uterus and the organism from the consequences of a pregnancy which it is not able to sustain. . . . In these cases the use of medication has as its end the prevention of conception by preventing ovulation. They are instances, therefore, of direct sterilization.

—Pius XII, "Morality and Eugenics," Address to the Participants in the Seventh Congress of the International Society of Hematology, September 12, 1958

61. Is a hysterectomy (i.e., removal of the uterus) or a tubal ligation (i.e., prevention of ovulation by blocking the fallopian tubes) permissible if the uterus is known to be incapable of carrying a future pregnancy to term?

The uterus as described . . . does not constitute in and of itself any present danger to the woman. . . . Therefore, the described procedures do not have a properly therapeutic character but are aimed in themselves at rendering sterile future sexual acts freely chosen. The end of avoiding risks to the mother, deriving from a possible pregnancy, is thus pursued by means of a direct sterilization, in itself always morally illicit, while other ways, which are morally licit, remain open to free choice.

—Congregation for the Doctrine of the Faith, *Responses to Questions Proposed Concerning "Uterine Isolation" and Related Matters*

62. Is a hysterectomy permissible if the uterus itself is seriously injured (e.g., uncontrolled hemorrhaging during a Caesarian section delivery) such that its removal prevents an immediate threat to the life or health of the mother?

EDITOR'S NOTE: The former question, number 61, is asking whether a sterilizing action is permissible if, without the hysterectomy or tubal ligation, human life would not survive (if conception were to occur). The present question concerns an emergent situation in which saving the life of the mother requires doing an action that has an unintended effect of sterilizing the mother—via removing the uterus.

In [this] case, the hysterectomy is licit because it has a directly therapeutic character, even though it may be foreseen that permanent sterility will result. In fact, it is the pathological condition of the uterus (e.g., a hemorrhage which cannot be stopped by other means), which makes its removal medically indicated. The removal of the organ has as its aim, therefore, the curtailing of a serious present danger to the woman independent of a possible future pregnancy.

—Congregation for the Doctrine of the Faith, *Responses to Questions Proposed Concerning "Uterine Isolation" and Related Matters*

63. Is a hysterectomy permissible if the uterus is functional enough for implantation, but not enough to tolerate gestation, namely, it cannot bear a child to the point of viability?

In the case considered in the question, it is known that the reproductive organs are not capable of protecting a conceived child up to viability, namely, they are not capable of fulfilling their natural procreative function. The objective of the procreative process is to bring a baby into the world, but here the birth of a living fetus is not biologically possible. Therefore, we are not dealing with a defective, or risky, functioning of the reproductive organs, but we are faced here with a situation in which the natural end of bringing a living child into the world is not attainable.

The medical procedure should not be judged as being against procreation, because we find ourselves within an objective context in which neither procreation, nor as a consequence, an anti-procreative action, are possible. Removing a reproductive organ incapable of bringing a pregnancy to term should not therefore be qualified as direct sterilization, which is and remains intrinsically illicit as an end and as a means.

—Congregation for the Doctrine of the Faith, *Response to a Question on the Liceity of a Hysterectomy in Certain Cases*

3

Genetics

64. Is prenatal diagnosis permissible?

Prenatal diagnosis, which presents no moral objections if carried out in order to identify the medical treatment which may be needed by the child in the womb, all too often becomes an opportunity for proposing and procuring an abortion. This is eugenic abortion, justified in public opinion on the basis of a mentality—mistakenly held to be consistent with the demands of "therapeutic interventions"—which accepts life only under certain conditions and rejects it when it is affected by any limitation, handicap, or illness.

—John Paul II, *Evangelium vitae*, 14

Such diagnosis is permissible, with the consent of the parents after they have been adequately informed, if the methods employed safeguard the life and integrity of the embryo and the mother, without subjecting them to disproportionate risks.

—Congregation for the Doctrine of the Faith, *Donum vitae*, I.2

The *purposes* for which prenatal diagnosis may be requested and performed must always be *for the benefit* of the child and of the mother, whether they are directed to the enabling of therapeutic interventions, to providing certainty and peace of mind to pregnant women who are anxious about the possibility of fetal malformations and are tempted to resort to abortion, or in the case of an unfavorable outcome, to preparing them to welcome the life of a child with a handicap.

—Pontifical Council for Pastoral Assistance to Health Care Workers,
New Charter for Health Care Workers, 35

Prenatal diagnosis is permitted when the procedure does not threaten the life or physical integrity of the unborn child or the mother and does not subject them to disproportionate risks; when the diagnosis can provide information to guide preventative care for the mother or pre- or postnatal care for the child; and when the parents, or at least the mother, give free and informed consent. Prenatal diagnosis is not permitted when undertaken with the intention of aborting an unborn child with a serious defect.

—USCCB, *Ethical and Religious Directives for Catholic Health Care Services*, 50

65. Are there circumstances when prenatal diagnosis would not be permissible?

[Prenatal diagnosis] is gravely opposed to the moral law when it is done with the thought of possibly inducing an abortion depending upon the results: a diagnosis which shows the existence of a malformation or a hereditary illness must not be the equivalent of a death sentence.

—Congregation for the Doctrine of the Faith, *Donum vitae*, I.2

The spouse or relatives or anyone else would similarly be acting in a manner contrary to the moral law if they were to counsel or impose such a diagnostic procedure on the expectant mother with the same intention of possibly proceeding to an abortion. So too the specialist would be guilty of illicit collaboration if, in conducting the diagnosis and in communicating its results, he were deliberately to contribute to establishing or favoring a link between prenatal diagnosis and abortion.

—Congregation for the Doctrine of the Faith, *Donum vitae*, I.2

The Catholic Church, which considers man redeemed by Christ as her way, insists that the recognition of the dignity of the human being as a person from the moment of conception also be guaranteed by law. Furthermore, she asks political leaders and scientists to promote the good of the person through scientific research aimed at perfecting appropriate treatments that are feasible and without disproportionate risks. This is possible, as scientists themselves acknowledge, in therapeutic interventions on the genome of somatic cells, but not on the genome of germinal cells and that of the premature embryo. I feel an obligation here to express my concern over the spread of a cultural climate which is steering prenatal diagnosis in a direction that is no longer one of treatment for the sake of better accepting the life of the unborn, but rather one of discrimination against those who do not prove healthy in

prenatal examination. At the current time there is a serious dispropor-
tion between diagnostic possibilities, which are progressively expanding,
and therapeutic possibilities, which are scarce: this fact raises serious
ethical problems for families, who need to be supported in welcoming
newborn life, even when it suffers from some defect or malformation.

In this regard, it is necessary to denounce the rise and spread of a
new selective eugenics, which leads to the suppression of embryos and
fetuses suffering from any disease. Sometimes baseless theories about
the anthropological and ethical difference of the various developmental
stages of prenatal life are employed: the so-called progressive humanization of the fetus. Sometimes an appeal is made to a mistaken idea of
the quality of life, which should—it is said—prevail over the sacredness
of life. In this regard, we cannot fail to ask that the rights proclaimed by
the conventions and international declarations on the protection of the
human genome and, in general, on the right to life be enjoyed by every
human being from the moment of fertilization, without any form of
discrimination, whether related to genetic imperfections or physical
defects, or to various stages of the human being's development. Therefore, it is urgently necessary to reinforce the legal bulwark in view of
the immense diagnostic possibilities brought to light by the project of
sequencing the human genome.

—John Paul II, Address to the Members of the
Pontifical Academy for Life, February 24, 1998, 5–6

66. Is genetic counseling permissible?

Genetic counseling may be provided in order to promote responsible parenthood and to prepare for the proper treatment and care of
children with genetic defects, in accordance with Catholic moral teaching and the intrinsic rights and obligations of married couples regarding
the transmission of life.

—USCCB, *Ethical and Religious Directives for Catholic Health Care Services*, 54

67. Is pre-implantation genetic diagnosis permissible?

[Preimplantation genetic diagnosis] involves the genetic diagnosis
of embryos that are engendered in vitro before they are transferred to
the uterus, in order to selectively use embryos without genetic defects or
with desired characteristics. Preimplantation genetic diagnosis is in fact

an expression of a eugenic mentality that legitimizes selective abortion to prevent the birth of babies afflicted with various illnesses.

—Pontifical Council for Pastoral Assistance to Health Care Workers, *New Charter for Health Care Workers*, 36

Preimplantation diagnosis is therefore the expression of a *eugenic mentality* that "accepts selective abortion in order to prevent the birth of children affected by various types of anomalies. Such an attitude is shameful and utterly reprehensible, since it presumes to measure the value of a human life only within the parameters of 'normality' and physical well-being, thus opening the way to legitimizing infanticide and euthanasia as well."

—Congregation for the Doctrine of the Faith, *Dignitas personae* 22 (quoting John Paul II, *Evangelium vitae*, 63)

68. Is enhancement of human capabilities or life extension through genetic manipulation permissible?

The biological nature of each person is untouchable in the sense that it is constitutive of the personal identity of the individual throughout the whole course of his history. Each human person, in his absolutely unique singularly, is constituted not only by his spirit, but by his body as well. Thus, in the body and through the body, one touches the person himself in his concrete reality. To respect the dignity of man consequently amounts to safeguarding this identity of the man "*corpore et anima unus*," as Vatican Council II says. It is on the basis of this anthropological vision that one should find the fundamental criteria for decision making in the case of not strictly therapeutic interventions, for example those aimed at the amelioration of the human biological condition.

In particular, this kind of intervention must not infringe on the origin of human life, that is, procreation linked to the union, not only biological but also spiritual, of the parents, united by the bond of marriage. It must consequently respect the fundamental dignity of man and the common biological nature which is at the base of liberty, avoiding manipulations that tend to modify genetic inheritance and to create groups of different men at the risk of causing new cases of marginalization in society.

Moreover, the fundamental attitudes that inspire the interventions of which we are speaking should not flow from a racist and materialist mentality aimed at a human well-being that is in reality reductionist. The dignity of man transcends his biological condition.

Genetic manipulation becomes arbitrary and unjust when it reduces life to an object, when it forgets that it is dealing with a human subject, capable of intelligence and freedom, worthy of respect whatever may be their limitations; or when it treats this person in terms of criteria not founded on the integral reality of the human person, at the risk of infringing upon his dignity. In this case, it exposes the individual to the caprice of others, thus depriving him of his autonomy.

—John Paul II, Address at the Conclusion of the Thirty-fifth General Assembly of the World Medical Association, October 29, 1983 (quoting Vatican Council II, *Gaudium et spes*, 14)

The question of using genetic engineering for purposes other than medical treatment also calls for consideration. Some have imagined the possibility of using techniques of genetic engineering to introduce alterations with the presumed aim of improving and strengthening the gene pool. Some of these proposals exhibit a certain dissatisfaction or even rejection of the value of the human being as a finite creature and person. Apart from technical difficulties and the real and potential risks involved, such manipulation would promote a eugenic mentality and would lead to indirect social stigma with regard to people who lack certain qualities, while privileging qualities that happen to be appreciated by a certain culture or society; such qualities do not constitute what is specifically human. This would be in contrast with the fundamental truth of the equality of all human beings which is expressed in the principle of justice, the violation of which, in the long run, would harm peaceful coexistence among individuals. Furthermore, one wonders who would be able to establish which modifications were to be held as positive and which not, or what limits should be placed on individual requests for improvement since it would be materially impossible to fulfil the wishes of every single person. Any conceivable response to these questions would, however, derive from arbitrary and questionable criteria. All of this leads to the conclusion that the prospect of such an intervention would end sooner or later by harming the common good, by favoring the will of some over the freedom of others. Finally it must also be noted that in the attempt to create *a new type of human being* one can recognize *an ideological element* in which man tries to take the place of his Creator.

In stating the ethical negativity of these kinds of interventions which imply *an unjust domination of man over man*, the Church also recalls the need to return to an attitude of care for people and of education in accepting human life in its concrete, historical, finite nature.

—Congregation for the Doctrine of the Faith, *Dignitas personae*, 27

4

The Body and Bodily Dimension of Sexual Love

69. What does the Church say about sex reassignment surgery?

EDITOR'S NOTE: Sex reassignment *surgery* involves at least two actions: in many cases, it removes healthy organs, i.e., male genitalia or breast tissue/areola for mastectomy; and in all cases it renders the patient sterile. ✢

Direct sterilization of either men or women, whether permanent or temporary, is not permitted in a Catholic healthcare institution.

—USCCB, *Ethical and Religious Directives for Catholic Health Care Services*, 53

All persons served by Catholic health care have the right and duty to protect and preserve their bodily and functional integrity.

—USCCB, *Ethical and Religious Directives for Catholic Health Care Services*, 29

According to ... scientific research, the human person is so profoundly affected by sexuality that it must be considered as one of the factors which give to each individual's life the principal traits that distinguish it. In fact it is from sex that the human person receives the characteristics which, on the biological, psychological, and spiritual levels, make that person a man or a woman, and thereby largely condition his or her progress towards maturity and insertion into society.

—Congregation for the Doctrine of the Faith, *Persona humana*, 1

Though made of body and soul, man is one. Through his bodily composition, he gathers to himself the elements of the material world; thus they reach their crown through him, and through him raise their voice in free praise of the Creator. For this reason man is not allowed to despise his bodily life, rather he is obliged to regard his body as good and honorable since God has created it and will raise it up on the last day. Nevertheless, wounded by sin, man experiences rebellious stirrings in his body. But the very dignity of man postulates that man glorify God in his body and forbid it to serve the evil inclinations of his heart.

—Vatican Council II, *Gaudium et spes*, 14

The spiritual and immortal soul is the principle of unity of the human being, whereby it exists as a whole—*corpore et anima unus*—as a person. . . . Reason and free will are linked with all the bodily and sense faculties. . . . The human person cannot be reduced to a freedom which is self-designing, but entails a particular spiritual and bodily structure.

—John Paul II, *Veritatis splendor*, 48

70. Are other forms of body modifications such as cosmetic surgery permissible?

EDITOR'S NOTE: There is no magisterial teaching that is explicitly directed to cosmetic surgery, but it is a question that many ask. Since most cosmetic surgeries do not frustrate normal human functioning, the ethical concern is not that it might violate the principle of totality (see above) or that it might count as a mutilation. At issue is whether cosmetic acts count as vainglorious. But even if this correctly identifies the abstract category of ethical concern, there is still room for much more precision. A fashion model whose job depends on maintaining a certain look may justifiably receive some cosmetic surgery—assuming a medically proportionate risk–benefit ratio. People use makeup or exercise (for other than health reasons), and there is no obvious ethical concern with such cosmetic actions either. In fact, trying to look good for one's spouse is not just permissible, but may be required by charity; the other feels respected and honored when a spouse tries to look his or her best for the other. Though these are not surgical actions, the point is that what counts as the capital vice of vainglory does not apply to much of what we do to care for our appearance. So, the importance of this question is that the answer should delineate the line between proper care for one's appearance versus vainglorious concern for or self-preoccupation with one's appearance. The following reflections from Saint Thomas Aquinas on vainglory, and the *Catechism of the Catholic Church* on the respect due to the body deserve attention but are not definitive answers. ✛

The desire for glory [i.e., to be known or recognized] does not, of itself, denote a sin: but the desire for empty or vain glory denotes a sin: for it is sinful to desire anything vain, according to Psalm 4:3, "Why do you love vanity, and seek after lying?"

Now glory may be called vain in three ways. First, on the part of the thing for which one seeks glory: as when a man seeks glory for that which is unworthy of glory, for instance when he seeks it for something frail and perishable; secondly, on the part of him from whom he seeks glory, for instance a man whose judgment is uncertain [The Latin is *non certum* which can mean not reliable or not fixed]; thirdly, on the part of the man himself who seeks glory, for that he does not refer the desire of his own glory to a due end, such as God's honor, or the spiritual welfare of his neighbor.

—Thomas Aquinas, *Summa theologiae*, II-II, q. 132, a. 1, resp.

If morality requires respect for the life of the body, it does not make it an absolute value. It rejects a neo-pagan notion that tends to promote the *cult of the body*, to sacrifice everything for its sake, to idolize physical perfection.

—*Catechism of the Catholic Church*, 2289

71. Is it moral to prescribe erectile dysfunction therapy to unmarried men?

EDITOR'S NOTE: This question concerns the extent to which the doctor would cooperate in the immoral acts of another (i.e., fornication, etc.). ✛

The cooperation is *material* if the one cooperating neither shares the wrongdoer's intention in performing the immoral act nor cooperates by directly participating in the act as a means to some other end, but rather contributes to the immoral activity in a way that is causally related but not essential to the immoral act itself.

—USCCB, *Ethical and Religious Directives for Catholic Health Care Services*, Part Six, introduction

Catholic healthcare organizations are not permitted to engage in immediate material cooperation in actions that are intrinsically immoral, such as abortion, euthanasia, assisted suicide, and direct sterilization.

—USCCB, *Ethical and Religious Directives for Catholic Health Care Services*, 70

Cooperation is formal not only when the cooperator shares the intention of the wrongdoer, but also when the cooperator directly participates in the immoral act, even if the cooperator does not share the intention of the wrongdoer, but participates as a means to some other end. Formal cooperation may take various forms, such as authorizing wrongdoing, approving it, prescribing it, actively defending it, or giving specific direction about carrying it out. Formal cooperation, in whatever form, is always morally wrong.

—USCCB, *Ethical and Religious Directives for Catholic Health Care Services*, Part Six, introduction

From the moral standpoint, it is never licit to cooperate formally in evil. Such cooperation occurs when an action, either by its very nature or by the form it takes in a concrete situation, can be defined as a direct participation in an act against innocent human life or a sharing in the immoral intention of the person committing it. This cooperation can never be justified either by invoking respect for the freedom of others or by appealing to the fact that civil law permits it or requires it. Each individual in fact has moral responsibility for the acts which he personally performs; no one can be exempted from this responsibility, and on the basis of it everyone will be judged by God himself.

—John Paul II, *Evangelium vitae*, 74

5

Vaccines and Vaccination

72. Does the Catholic Church recommend vaccination?

From the perspective of preventing infectious diseases, the development of vaccines and their employment in the fight against such infections, through the obligatory immunization of all the populations concerned, is undoubtedly a positive step.

—Pontifical Council for Pastoral Assistance to Health Care Workers, *New Charter for Health Care Workers*, 69

73. Is it permissible for *a researcher* to develop drugs or vaccines using cell lines derived from aborted fetuses?

According to this criterion [the criterion of independence], the use of "biological material" of illicit origin would be ethically permissible provided there is a clear separation between those who, on the one hand, produce, freeze, and cause the death of embryos and, on the other, the researchers involved in scientific experimentation. The criterion of independence is not sufficient to avoid a contradiction in the attitude of the person who says that he does not approve of the injustice perpetrated by others, but at the same time accepts for his own work the "biological material" which the others have obtained by means of that injustice. When the illicit action is endorsed by the laws which regulate healthcare and scientific research, it is necessary to distance oneself from the evil aspects of that system in order not to give the impression of a certain toleration or tacit acceptance of actions which are gravely unjust. Any appearance of acceptance would in fact contribute to the growing indifference to, if not the approval of, such actions in certain medical and political circles.

—Congregation for the Doctrine of the Faith, *Dignitas personae*, 35

74. Is it permissible for *a person/patient* to receive a vaccine developed and/or tested on cell lines that were derived from aborted fetal tissue?

Within this general picture there exist *differing degrees of responsibility*. Grave reasons may be morally proportionate to justify the use of such "biological material." Thus, for example, danger to the health of children could permit parents to use a vaccine which was developed using cell lines of illicit origin, while keeping in mind that everyone has the duty to make known their disagreement and to ask that their healthcare system make other types of vaccines available.

—Congregation for the Doctrine of the Faith, *Dignitas personae*, 35

The fundamental reason for considering the use of these vaccines morally licit is that the kind of cooperation in evil (*passive material cooperation*) in the procured abortion from which these cell lines originate is, on the part of those making use of the resulting vaccines, *remote*. The moral duty to avoid such passive material cooperation is not obligatory if there is a grave danger, such as the otherwise uncontainable spread of a serious pathological agent.

—Congregation for the Doctrine of the Faith, *Note on the Morality of Using Some Anti-COVID-19 Vaccines*, 3

6

At the End of Life

A Plea for Love

75. What does the Church say about euthanasia and physician-assisted suicide?

EDITOR'S NOTE: The two actions are similar except that for euthanasia the doctor is the agent who brings about the patient's death, and for physician-assisted suicide, the doctor prescribes a lethal cocktail of drugs with the intention that the patient commit suicide with them. The latter is formal cooperation, see above, in the evil of someone's suicide, the former is a case of intentional killing. ✢

In order that the question of euthanasia can be properly dealt with, it is first necessary to define the words used.

Etymologically speaking, in ancient times *euthanasia* meant an *easy death* without severe suffering. Today one no longer thinks of this original meaning of the word, but rather of some intervention of medicine whereby the suffering of sickness or of the final agony are reduced, sometimes also with the danger of suppressing life prematurely. Ultimately, the word *euthanasia* is used in a more particular sense to mean "mercy killing," for the purpose of putting an end to extreme suffering, or saving abnormal babies, the mentally ill, or the incurably sick from the prolongation, perhaps for many years of a miserable life, which could impose too heavy a burden on their families or on society.

It is, therefore, necessary to state clearly in what sense the word is used in the present document.

By euthanasia is understood an action or an omission which of itself or by intention causes death, in order that all suffering may in this way be eliminated. Euthanasia's terms of reference, therefore, are to be found in the intention of the will and in the methods used.

It is necessary to state firmly once more that nothing and no one can in any way permit the killing of an innocent human being, whether a fetus or an embryo, an infant or an adult, an old person, or one suffering from an incurable disease, or a person who is dying. Furthermore, no one is permitted to ask for this act of killing, either for himself or herself or for another person entrusted to his or her care, nor can he or she consent to it, either explicitly or implicitly. Nor can any authority legitimately recommend or permit such an action. For it is a question of the violation of the divine law, an offense against the dignity of the human person, a crime against life, and an attack on humanity.

It may happen that, by reason of prolonged and barely tolerable pain, for deeply personal or other reasons, people may be led to believe that they can legitimately ask for death or obtain it for others. Although in these cases the guilt of the individual may be reduced or completely absent, nevertheless the error of judgment into which the conscience falls, perhaps in good faith, does not change the nature of this act of killing, which will always be in itself something to be rejected. The pleas of gravely ill people who sometimes ask for death are not to be understood as implying a true desire for euthanasia; in fact, it is almost always a case of an anguished plea for help and love. What a sick person needs, besides medical care, is love, the human and supernatural warmth with which the sick person can and ought to be surrounded by all those close to him or her, parents and children, doctors and nurses.

—Congregation for the Doctrine of the Faith,
Declaration on Euthanasia, II

Each life has the same value and dignity for everyone: the respect of the life of another is the same as the respect owed to one's own life. One who choses with full liberty to take one's own life breaks one's relationship with God and with others, and renounces oneself as a moral subject. Assisted suicide aggravates the gravity of this act because it implicates another in one's own despair. Another person is led to turn his will from the mystery of God in the theological virtue of hope and thus to repudiate the authentic value of life and to break the covenant that establishes the human family. Assisting in a suicide is an unjustified collaboration in an unlawful act that contradicts the theological relationship with God and the moral relationship that unites us with others who share the gift of life and the meaning of existence.

—Congregation for the Doctrine of the Faith, *Samaritanus bonus*, V, 1

76. How does the Church view physician-assisted suicide in the context of it being legal in some US states or other countries?

The doctrine on the necessary *conformity of civil law with the moral law* is in continuity with the whole tradition of the Church. This is clear once more from John XXIII's encyclical: "Authority is a postulate of the moral order and derives from God. Consequently, laws and decrees enacted in contravention of the moral order, and hence of the divine will, can have no binding force in conscience. . . ; indeed, the passing of such laws undermines the very nature of authority and results in shameful abuse" (*Pacem in terris*, II). This is the clear teaching of Saint Thomas Aquinas, who writes that "human law is law inasmuch as it is in conformity with right reason and thus derives from the eternal law. But when a law is contrary to reason, it is called an unjust law; but in this case it ceases to be a law and becomes instead an act of violence" (*Summa theologiae*, I-II, q. 93, a. 3, ad 2). And again: "Every law made by man can be called a law insofar as it derives from the natural law. But if it is somehow opposed to the natural law, then it is not really a law but rather a corruption of the law" (*Summa theologiae*, I-II, q. 95, a. 2).

Now the first and most immediate application of this teaching concerns a human law which disregards the fundamental right and source of all other rights which is the right to life, a right belonging to every individual. Consequently, laws which legitimize the direct killing of innocent human beings through abortion or euthanasia are in complete opposition to the inviolable right to life proper to every individual; they thus deny the equality of everyone before the law. It might be objected that such is not the case in euthanasia, when it is requested with full awareness by the person involved. But any State which made such a request legitimate and authorized it to be carried out would be legalizing a case of suicide-murder, contrary to the fundamental principles of absolute respect for life and of the protection of every innocent life. In this way the State contributes to lessening respect for life and opens the door to ways of acting which are destructive of trust in relations between people. Laws which authorize and promote abortion and euthanasia are therefore radically opposed not only to the good of the individual but also to the common good; as such they are completely lacking in authentic juridical validity. Disregard for the right to life, precisely because it leads to the killing of the person whom society exists to serve, is what most directly conflicts with the possibility of achieving the common good.

Consequently, a civil law authorizing abortion or euthanasia ceases by that very fact to be a true, morally binding civil law.

—John Paul II, *Evangelium vitae*, 72

In the face of the legalization of euthanasia or assisted suicide—even when viewed simply as another form of medical assistance—formal or immediate material cooperation must be excluded. Such situations offer specific occasions for Christian witness where "we must obey God rather than men" (Acts 5:29). There is no right to suicide nor to euthanasia: laws exist, not to cause death, but to protect life and to facilitate co-existence among human beings. It is therefore never morally lawful to collaborate with such immoral actions or to imply collusion in word, action, or omission. The one authentic right is that the sick person be accompanied and cared for with genuine humanity. Only in this way can the patient's dignity be preserved until the moment of natural death.

—Congregation for the Doctrine of the Faith, *Samaritanus bonus*, V, 9

Moral Obligations and Options

77. Is it ever morally acceptable to withhold life-sustaining medical care? Does being pro-life mean always fighting against death with all available medical tools?

Euthanasia must be distinguished from the decision to forgo so-called aggressive medical treatment, in other words, medical procedures which no longer correspond to the real situation of the patient, either because they are by now disproportionate to any expected results or because they impose an excessive burden on the patient and his family. In such situations, when death is clearly imminent and inevitable, one can in conscience "refuse forms of treatment that would only secure a precarious and burdensome prolongation of life, so long as the normal care due to the sick person in similar cases is not interrupted." Certainly, there is a moral obligation to care for oneself and to allow oneself to be cared for, but this duty must take account of concrete circumstances. It needs to be determined whether the means of treatment available are objectively proportionate to the prospects for improvement. To forgo extraordinary or disproportionate means is not the equivalent of suicide or euthanasia; it rather expresses acceptance of the human condition in the face of death.

—John Paul II, *Evangelium vitae*, 65 (quoting Congregation for the Doctrine of the Faith, *Declaration on Euthanasia*, IV)

If recovery is impossible, the healthcare worker must never give up taking care of the person.[1] He is obliged to provide all *ordinary and proportionate care*.

Care is to be considered proportionate when there is *due proportion* between the means employed and therapeutic effectiveness. To verify this due proportion, one must "make a correct judgment as to the means by studying the type of treatment to be used, its degree of complexity or risk, its cost, and the possibilities of using it, and comparing these elements with the result that can be expected, taking into account the state of the sick person and his or her physical and moral resources."

Means are to be considered *extraordinary*, on the other hand, when they impose a heavy or excessive burden (whether material, physical, moral, or economic) on the patient, his family members, or the health-care institution. With all the more reason, treatments that have become futile must not be continued.

The use of *ordinary means* of sustaining the patient's life is morally obligatory. On the other hand, extraordinary means may be declined with the patient's consent or upon his request, even if this hastens death. Physicians cannot be obliged to employ extraordinary means.

—Pontifical Council for Pastoral Assistance to Health Care Workers, *New Charter for Health Care Workers*, 86 (quoting Congregation for the Doctrine of the Faith, *Declaration on Euthanasia*, IV)

78. How should one understand the principle of the *proportionality of treatment* just mentioned?

If there are no other sufficient remedies, it is permitted, with the patient's consent, to have recourse to the means provided by the most advanced medical techniques, even if these means are still at the experimental stage and are not without a certain risk.

---

1 Note from *New Charter for Health Care Workers*, 86: "Even when it cannot cure, science can and must care for and assist the patient" (John Paul II, Address to participants in a course on human pre-leukemias, November 15, 1985), 5.

It is also permitted, with the patient's consent, to interrupt these means, where the results fall short of expectations. But for such a decision to be made, account will have to be taken of the reasonable wishes of the patient and the patient's family, as also of the advice of the doctors who are specially competent in the matter. The latter may in particular judge that the investment in instruments and personnel is disproportionate to the results foreseen; they may also judge that the techniques applied impose on the patient strain or suffering out of proportion with the benefits which he or she may gain from such techniques.

It is also permissible to make do with the normal means that medicine can offer. Therefore one cannot impose on anyone the obligation to have recourse to a technique which is already in use but which carries a risk or is burdensome. Such a refusal is not the equivalent of suicide; on the contrary, it should be considered as an acceptance of the human condition, or a wish to avoid the application of a medical procedure disproportionate to the results that can be expected, or a desire not to impose excessive expense on the family or the community.

—Congregation for the Doctrine of the Faith,
Declaration on Euthanasia, IV

79. What does "too burdensome" mean? Does it mean that the person is too much of a burden on their friends, family, or society?

["Too burdensome" means,] first, and most obviously, the fact that the only available treatments prove incapable of achieving the goal one had set out to achieve for a particular patient. The treatments one has tried (or perhaps merely contemplated) appear to be clearly futile.

Secondly, the treatments one contemplates or tries, though they may promise some medical benefit, in the sense of securing one of the goals of medicine, will impose grave burdens on the patient in doing so. These burdens may be unacceptable either because, independently of other considerations, they are excessively difficult to bear, or because bearing them does not seem warranted by the amount of benefit the treatment promises.

Sometimes, since the extent to which certain side effects are burdensome will depend very much on the dispositions and circumstances of the patient, one needs evidence (directly from the competent patient, or by way of testimony from those close to an incompetent patient) about those dispositions and circumstances in order to assess the extent to which what will be experienced as burdensome will be warranted by the likely benefits of treatment.

We should allow a wide interpretation to the notion of "burdens of treatment": they may be physical (as in pain); psychological (as in mental distress); social (as in disruption of life-style); and economic (as in the financial burdens they impose on others). But this wide interpretation of the scope of the notion of burden should be combined with a strict interpretation of what is meant by talking of "the burdens of treatment." "Burdens of treatment" means: burdens caused by treatment. A patient's life is not caused by his treatment, even though it may be true to say that a patient is enabled to stay alive through treatment. So survival with disability should not be counted among the burdens of treatment. If it is, and if it is regarded as a reason for ceasing treatment, then you make the aim of ceasing treatment to be that of putting an end to the existence of the patient.

On the other hand, the fact that a person is disabled in a particular way may make it predictable that a particular course of treatment will be excessively burdensome. Disability can be relevant in that way to a reasonable decision to withhold some course of treatment. This illustrates one way in which a particular type of "quality-of-life" judgement is relevant to decisions to withhold and withdraw treatment. The type of judgement in question is one which focuses on the condition of the patient as that is relevant to assessing the prospective benefits and burdens of treatment. One's interest is in determining those benefits and burdens. There is a quite distinct kind of quality-of-life judgement for which the focus is not on the worthwhileness of treatment, as one may assess that in terms of its benefits and burdens, but rather on the worthwhileness of the patient's life. As we have already seen, to shift focus in that way is already to have embarked on a potentially euthanasiast line of reasoning. To engage in judgements of that kind is incompatible with recognizing the dignity of the patient and his or her entitlement to just treatment. It is precisely such judgements, unfortunately, that the BMA's [British Medical Association] Consultation Paper envisages (at 2.9.7 and 2.11, no. 7) as the appropriate basis for withdrawing and withholding treatment in certain types of case.

Thirdly, one may be prevented from aiming at what one regards as an appropriate medical goal in the care of a patient by the competent patient's refusal of the relevant treatment. The veto power of competent patients may be exercised on the basis of good or bad reasons. Here we can take note of one kind of good reason which does not involve either futility or burdensomeness. In the following section we will clarify why bad reasons for refusing treatment are [a] reasonably allowed effect in the life of a competent patient, but should not be allowed [to be a] continuing effect when that once competent patient has become incompetent.

A competent patient may have good reason to refuse potentially beneficial treatment not because of any burdens consequent upon treatment but because other obligations stand in the way of the patient undergoing treatment. Clearly it is down to the competent patient to say whether this is the case, and there could be no moral justification for a doctor seeking to prevent a patient discharging overriding moral obligations.

Finally, one may be prevented from aiming at an appropriate medical goal by resource constraints: personnel, facilities, equipment, or medication are not available.

—Anscombe Bioethics Centre, Response to
Withdrawing and Withholding Treatment, 3.2

EDITOR'S NOTE: As noted in the introduction, selections outside of the magisterial framework were chosen if they satisfied one or all the following criteria: (i) There is no direct teaching on the matter by the Magisterium; (ii) The guidance given reflects the mind of the Church even if not formally taught; (iii) The guidance given is directly relevant and informative. We believe that this quotation, though lengthy, satisfies all three: there is no direct teaching on what counts as a burden, the guidance is ethically consistent with the mind of the Church, and it is informative because it gives specifics. ✢

80. What is the Church's view on choosing a do not resuscitate (DNR) order, or forgoing other forms of potentially life-sustaining therapies?

Natural reason and Christian morality say that man (and anyone who is charged with caring for his fellow man) has the right and duty, in the event of serious illness, to take the necessary measures to preserve life and health. Such a duty that he has to himself, to God, to the human community, and most often to determined people, derives from well-ordered charity, submission to the Creator, social justice, and even strict justice, as well as piety toward the family.

But it usually obliges only the use of ordinary means (according to the circumstances of people, places, times, culture), that is, means that do not impose any extraordinary burden on oneself or on another. A more severe obligation would be too heavy for most men and would make it more difficult to acquire more important higher goods. Life, health, all temporal activity are indeed subordinated to spiritual ends. On the other hand, it is not forbidden to do more than is strictly necessary to preserve life and health, provided that you do not fail in more serious duties.

—Pius XII, Speech on Three Questions of Medical Morality Related to Resuscitation, November 24, 1957

The physician is not the lord of life, but neither is he the conqueror of death. *Death is an inevitable fact of human life, and the use of means for avoiding it must take into account the human condition.*

—John Paul II, Address to the Pontifical Academy of Sciences, October 21, 1985, 5

When inevitable death is imminent in spite of the means used, it is permitted in conscience to take the decision to refuse forms of treatment that would only secure a precarious and burdensome prolongation of life, so long as the normal care due to the sick person in similar cases is not interrupted.

—Congregation for the Doctrine of the Faith, *Declaration on Euthanasia*, IV

Forgoing these [potentially life-sustaining] treatments, which would only procure a tenuous and painful prolongation of life, can also indicate respect for the dying person's will, expressed in *statements or advance directives* concerning treatment, while excluding any act of euthanasia.

The patient may express in advance his will concerning the treatments to which he would or would not wish to be subjected in a case where, over the course of his sickness or because of unexpected trauma, he is no longer capable of expressing his own consent or disagreement.

—Pontifical Council for Pastoral Assistance to Health Care Workers, *New Charter for Health Care Workers*, 150

With her mission to transmit to the faithful the grace of the Redeemer and the holy law of God already discernible in the precepts of the natural moral law, the Church is obliged to intervene in order to exclude once again all ambiguity in the teaching of the Magisterium concerning euthanasia and assisted suicide, even where these practices have been legalized.

In particular, the dissemination of medical end-of-life protocols such as the Do Not Resuscitate Order or the Physician Orders for Life Sustaining Treatment—with all of their variations depending on national laws and contexts—were initially thought of as instruments to avoid aggressive medical treatment in the terminal phases of life. Today these protocols cause serious problems regarding the duty to protect the life of patients in the most critical stages of sickness. On the one hand, medical staff feel increasingly bound by the self-determination expressed in patient declarations that deprive physicians of their freedom and duty to safeguard life even where they could do so. On the other hand, in some healthcare settings, concerns have recently arisen about the widely reported abuse of such protocols viewed in a euthanistic perspective with the result that neither patients nor families are consulted in final decisions about care. This happens above all in the countries where, with the legalization of euthanasia, wide margins of ambiguity are left open in end-of-life law regarding the meaning of obligations to provide care.

—Congregation for the Doctrine of the Faith, *Samaritanus bonus*, V, 1

81. Is it morally licit to withhold or withdraw medically assisted nutrition and hydration?

The sick person in a vegetative state, awaiting recovery or a natural end, still has the right to basic health care (nutrition, hydration, cleanliness, warmth, etc.), and to the prevention of complications related to his confinement to bed. He also has the right to appropriate rehabilitative care and to be monitored for clinical signs of eventual recovery.

I should like particularly to underline how the administration of water and food, even when provided by artificial means, always represents a *natural means* of preserving life, not a *medical act*. Its use, furthermore, should be considered, in principle, *ordinary and proportionate*, and as such morally obligatory, insofar as and until it is seen to have attained its proper finality, which in the present case consists in providing nourishment to the patient and alleviation of his suffering.

The obligation to provide the "normal care due to the sick in such cases" includes, in fact, the use of nutrition and hydration. The evaluation of probabilities, founded on waning hopes for recovery when the vegetative state is prolonged beyond a year, cannot ethically justify the cessation or interruption of *minimal care* for the patient, including nutrition and hydration. Death by starvation or dehydration is, in fact, the only possible outcome as a result of their withdrawal. In this sense it ends up becoming, if done knowingly and willingly, true and proper euthanasia by omission.

—John Paul II, Address to the Participants in the International Congress on "Life-Sustaining Treatments and Vegetative State: Scientific Advances and Ethical Dilemmas," March 20, 2004, 4 (quoting Congregation for the Doctrine of the Faith, *Declaration on Euthanasia*, IV)

In principle, there is an obligation to provide patients with food and water, including medically assisted nutrition and hydration for those who cannot take food orally. This obligation extends to patients in chronic and presumably irreversible conditions (e.g., the "persistent vegetative state") who can reasonably be expected to live indefinitely if given such care. Medically assisted nutrition and hydration become morally optional when they cannot reasonably be expected to prolong life or when they would be "excessively burdensome for the patient or [would] cause significant physical discomfort, for example resulting from complications in the use of the means employed." For instance, as a patient draws close to inevitable death from an underlying progressive and fatal condition, certain measures to provide nutrition and hydration may become excessively burdensome and therefore not obligatory in light of their very limited ability to prolong life or provide comfort.

—USCCB, *Ethical and Religious Directives for Catholic Health Care Services*, 58 (quoting Congregation for the Doctrine of the Faith, Commentary on "Responses to Certain Questions of the United States Conference of Catholic Bishops Concerning Artificial Nutrition and Hydration")

82. Is palliative care a morally acceptable form of medical care?

A sick person in the terminal stage of his illness should receive all forms of care that allow for alleviation of the painfulness of the dying process. These correspond to so-called palliative care, which together with care for his physical, psychological, and spiritual needs, tends to create a *loving presence* around the dying person and his family members.

—Pontifical Council for Pastoral Assistance to Health Care Workers, *New Charter for Health Care Workers*, 147

It should be recognized, however, that the definition of palliative care has in recent years taken on a sometimes equivocal connotation. In some countries, national laws regulating palliative care (Palliative Care

Act) as well as the laws on the "end of life" (End-of-Life Law) provide, along with palliative treatments, something called Medical Assistance to the Dying (MAiD) that can include the possibility of requesting euthanasia and assisted suicide. Such legal provisions are a cause of grave cultural confusion: by including under palliative care the provision of integrated medical assistance for a voluntary death, they imply that it would be morally lawful to request euthanasia or assisted suicide.

In addition, palliative interventions to reduce the suffering of gravely or terminally ill patients in these regulatory contexts can involve the administration of medications that intend to hasten death, as well as the suspension or interruption of hydration and nutrition even when death is not imminent. In fact, such practices are equivalent to a *direct action or omission to bring about death and are therefore unlawful.* The growing diffusion of such legislation and of scientific guidelines of national and international professional societies, constitutes a socially irresponsible threat to many people, including a growing number of vulnerable persons who needed only to be better cared for and comforted but are instead being led to choose euthanasia and suicide.

—Congregation for the Doctrine of the Faith, *Samaritanus bonus*, V, 4

83. Is it immoral for a physician or nurse to administer a high dose of a narcotic medication to a patient in pain even if the dose of the medication hastens the patient's death?

In the terminal stage, high doses of analgesics may sometimes be necessary to alleviate pain; this entails the risk of collateral effects and complications, including the *hastening of death.* It is necessary, therefore, that analgesics be prescribed prudently and *according to the standards of the art.*

—Pontifical Council for Pastoral Assistance to Health Care Workers,
New Charter for Health Care Workers, 154

The use of painkillers to alleviate the sufferings of the dying, even at the risk of shortening their days, can be morally in conformity with human dignity if death is not willed as either an end or a means, but only foreseen and tolerated as inevitable.

—*Catechism of the Catholic Church,* 2279

In the presence of unbearable pain that is resistant to typical pain-management therapies, if the moment of death is near or if there are good reasons for anticipating a particular crisis at the moment of death, a serious clinical indication can involve, with the sick person's consent, the administration of drugs that cause a loss of consciousness.

This deep palliative sedation in the terminal stage, when clinically motivated, can be morally acceptable provided that it is done with the patient's consent, that appropriate information is given to the family members, that any intention of euthanasia is ruled out, and that the patient has been able to perform his moral, familial, and religious duties.

—Pontifical Council for Pastoral Assistance to Health Care Workers,
New Charter for Health Care Workers, 155

In modern medicine, increased attention is being given to what are called "methods of palliative care," which seek to make suffering more bearable in the final stages of illness and to ensure that the patient is supported and accompanied in his or her ordeal. Among the questions which arise in this context is that of the licitness of using various types of painkillers and sedatives for relieving the patient's pain when this involves the risk of shortening life. While praise may be due to the person who voluntarily accepts suffering by forgoing treatment with painkillers in order to remain fully lucid and, if a believer, to share consciously in the Lord's Passion, such "heroic" behavior cannot be considered the duty of everyone. Pius XII affirmed that it is licit to relieve pain by narcotics, even when the result is decreased consciousness and a shortening of life, "if no other means exist, and if, in the given circumstances, this does not prevent the carrying out of other religious and moral duties." In such a case, death is not willed or sought, even though for reasonable motives one runs the risk of it: there is simply a desire to ease pain effectively by using the analgesics which medicine provides. All the same, "it is not right to deprive the dying person of consciousness without a serious reason": as they approach death people ought to be able to satisfy their moral and family duties, and above all they ought to be able to prepare in a fully conscious way for their definitive meeting with God.

—John Paul II, *Evangelium vitae*, 65 (quoting Pius XII, Address
to an International Group of Physicians, February 24, 1957)

Organ Donation

84. What is the Church's view of organ transplantation?

Among the many remarkable achievements of modern medicine, advances in the fields of immunology and of surgical technology have made possible the therapeutic use of organ and tissue transplants. It is surely a reason for satisfaction that many sick people, who until recently could only expect death or at best a painful and restricted existence, can now recover more or less fully through the replacement of a diseased organ with a healthy donated one. We should rejoice that *medicine, in its service to life, has found in organ transplantation a new way of serving the human family*, precisely by safeguarding that fundamental good of the person.

This splendid development is not of course without its dark side. There is still much to be learned through research and clinical experience, and there are *many questions of an ethical, legal, and social nature which need to be more deeply and widely investigated.* There are even shameful abuses which call for determined action on the part of medical associations and donor societies, and especially of competent legislative bodies. Yet in spite of these difficulties, we can recall the words of the fourth-century Doctor of the Church, Saint Basil the Great: "As regards medicine, it would not be right to reject a gift of God (that is, medical science), just because of the bad use that some people make of it . . . ; we should instead throw light on what they have corrupted."

With the advent of organ transplantation, which began with blood transfusions, man has found a way to give of himself, of his blood and of his body, so that others may continue to live. Thanks to science, and to the professional training and commitment of doctors and healthcare workers, whose collaboration is less obvious but no less indispensable for the outcome of complicated surgical operations, new and wonderful challenges are presented. We are challenged to love our neighbor in new ways; in evangelical terms, to love "to the end" (Cf. Jn 13:1), yet within certain limits which cannot be exceeded, limits laid down by human nature itself.

—John Paul II, Address to Participants of the First International Congress of the Society for Organ Sharing, June 20, 1991, 1–2 (quoting St. Basil the Great, *Regola lunga*)

85. What does the Church say about organ donation?

Above all, this form of treatment is inseparable from a *human act of donation*. In effect, transplantation presupposes a prior, explicit, free, and conscious decision on the part of the donor or of someone who legitimately represents the donor, generally the closest relatives. It is a decision to offer, without reward, a part of one's own body for the health and well-being of another person. In this sense, the medical action of transplantation makes possible the donor's act of self-giving, that sincere gift of self which expresses our constitutive calling to love and communion.

Love, communion, solidarity, and absolute respect for the dignity of the human person constitute the only legitimate context of organ transplantation. It is essential not to ignore the moral and spiritual values which come into play when individuals, while observing the ethical norms which guarantee the dignity of the human person and bring it to perfection, freely and consciously decide to give a part of themselves, a part of their own body, in order to save the life of another human being.

In effect, the human body is always a personal body, the body of a person. The body cannot be treated as a merely physical or biological entity, nor can its organs and tissues ever be used as items for sale or exchange. Such a reductive materialist conception would lead to a merely instrumental use of the body, and therefore of the person. In such a perspective, organ transplantation and the grafting of tissue would no longer correspond to an act of donation but would amount to the dispossession or plundering of a body.

Furthermore, a person can only donate that of which he can deprive himself without serious danger or harm to his own life or personal identity, and for a just and proportionate reason. It is obvious that vital organs can only be donated *after death*. But to offer in life a part of one's body, an offering which will become effective only after death, is already in many cases an act of *great love*, the love which gives life to others.

Thus the progress of the bio-medical sciences has made it possible for people to project beyond death their vocation to love. By analogy with Christ's Paschal Mystery, in dying death is somehow overcome and life [restored].

—John Paul II, Address to Participants of the First International Congress of the Society for Organ Sharing, June 20, 1991, 3–4

86. What has the Church said about "brain death"?

It is a well-known fact that for some time certain scientific approaches to ascertaining death have shifted the emphasis from the traditional cardio-respiratory signs to the so-called neurological criterion. Specifically, this consists in establishing, according to clearly determined parameters commonly held by the international scientific community, the complete and irreversible cessation of all brain activity (in the cerebrum, cerebellum, and brain stem). This is then considered the sign that the individual organism has lost its integrative capacity.

With regard to the parameters used today for ascertaining death— whether the "encephalic" signs or the more traditional cardio-respiratory signs—the Church does not make technical decisions. She limits herself to the Gospel duty of comparing the data offered by medical science with the Christian understanding of the unity of the person, bringing out the similarities and the possible conflicts capable of endangering respect for human dignity.

Here it can be said that the criterion adopted in more recent times for ascertaining the fact of death, namely the *complete* and *irreversible* cessation of all brain activity, if rigorously applied, does not seem to conflict with the essential elements of a sound anthropology. Therefore a health worker professionally responsible for ascertaining death can use these criteria in each individual case as the basis for arriving at that degree of assurance in ethical judgement which moral teaching describes as "moral certainty." This moral certainty is considered the necessary and sufficient basis for an ethically correct course of action. Only where such certainty exists, and where informed consent has already been given by the donor or the donor's legitimate representatives, is it morally right to initiate the technical procedures required for the removal of organs for transplant.

—John Paul II, Address to the Eighteenth International Congress
of the Transplantation Society, August 29, 2000, 5

87. Would a brain transplant, should this someday be possible, be morally acceptable?

Not all organs can be donated. From the ethical perspective, the brain and the gonads are ruled out as potential transplants, inasmuch as they are connected respectively with the *personal and procreative identity of the person.* These are organs specifically connected with the uniqueness of the person, which medicine must safeguard.

—Pontifical Council for Pastoral Assistance to Health Care Workers,
New Charter for Health Care Workers, 119

88. Is it morally permissible for a child to donate organs?

Particular care must be used in the *procurement of organs from pediatric donors* because of the need to apply to the child specifically tailored parameters for determining death and because of the delicate psychological situation of the parents, who are called upon to give consent for the removal. The need for organs from pediatric donors can in no way justify the omission of the proper verification of the clinical signs for the determination of death of a pediatric patient.

—Pontifical Council for Pastoral Assistance to Health Care Workers,
New Charter for Health Care Workers, 117

89. Is it morally permissible to accept tissue or organ transplantation from non-human sources?

There is an ongoing discussion about the possibility, which is still entirely experimental, of solving the problem of obtaining organs for human transplantation by resorting to the use of xenograft transplants, that is, *the transplantation of organs and tissues derived from animals.* "For a xenotransplant to be licit, the transplanted organ must not impair the integrity of the psychological or genetic identity of the person receiving it; and there must also be a proven biological possibility that the transplant will be successful and will not expose the recipient to inordinate risk." Moreover, it is necessary to respect the animals involved in these procedures by observing certain conditions: "Unnecessary animal suffering must be prevented; criteria of real necessity and reasonableness must be respected; genetic modifications that could significantly alter the biodiversity and the balance of the species in the animal world must be avoided."

—Pontifical Council for Pastoral Assistance to Health Care Workers,
New Charter for Health Care Workers, 118 (quoting John Paul II, Address to the
Eighteenth International Congress of the Transplantation Society, August 29,
2000, 7; and Pontifical Academy for Life, *Prospects for Xenotransplantation:
Scientific Aspects and Ethical Considerations,* 9)

Care for the Body after Death

90. What are guidelines for respecting the body after death with respect to autopsy, use for medical research, and education?

With respect to the question of removing a dead man's bodily parts to further therapeutic objectives, no doctor should be given the right to do with a corpse as he pleases. It is up to public authority to enact appropriate legislation regarding such matters. But public authority, on the other hand, does not have the right to proceed arbitrarily. There are certain provisions of the law to which it is possible to have serious objections. A norm, such as that which would permit a doctor in a sanatorium to remove parts of a body for therapeutic purposes—all thought of personal profit being duly forsworn—cannot be honored because of the existent possibility that it might be interpreted too freely. Then, too, the rights and duties of those whose obligation it is to assume responsibility for the body of the deceased must also be taken into consideration. And, finally, the demands of natural morality, which forbid us to consider and treat the body of a human being merely as a thing, or as that of an animal, must at all times be dutifully respected.

—Pius XII, Address to Participants in the Eighth Congress
of the World Medical Association, September 30, 1954

The public must be educated. It must be explained with intelligence and respect that to consent explicitly or tacitly to serious damage to the integrity of the corpse in the interest of those who are suffering, is no violation of the reverence due to the dead.

—Pius XII, Allocution to a Group of Eye Surgeons, May 14, 1956

Autopsies can be morally permitted for legal inquests or scientific research. The free gift of organs after death is legitimate and can be meritorious.

—*Catechism of the Catholic Church*, 2301

91. Is the Church against cremation?

Deceased members of the Christian faithful must be given ecclesiastical funerals according to the norm of law.

Ecclesiastical funerals, by which the Church seeks spiritual support for the deceased, honors their bodies, and at the same time brings the solace of hope to the living, must be celebrated according to the norm of the liturgical laws.

The Church earnestly recommends that the pious custom of burying the bodies of the deceased be observed; nevertheless, the Church does not prohibit cremation unless it was chosen for reasons contrary to Christian doctrine.

—*Code of Canon Law*, c. 1176 §3

In a letter dated November 16, 1966, the Reverend N.N., the chaplain of Evangelical Deaconess Hospital in the city of Cleveland, proposed to this Sacred Congregation two questions for which he sought a solution.

a) Whether it is licit for Catholics, of their own free will, to order that their own amputated members or those of others, as well as notable sections that are cut out [of the human body] be cremated, even apart from circumstances surrounding the case in which cremation would be imposed by medical or social reasons.

b) Fetus which have not completed 17 weeks of gestation—many of which are baptized—and notable parts of the human body are rarely buried but are usually cremated.

Is this practice intrinsically to be reprobated according to the fundamental principles of morality?

I inform you that the Fathers of this Sacred Congregation examined the questions proposed and, in the Plenary Session on Wednesday, the 1st of March of this year, decreed:

If there is a reasonable cause present which does not permit the burial of a fetus or member of the human body, there is no objection on the part of the Sacred Congregation for the Doctrine of the Faith to cremation.

—Congregation for the Doctrine of Faith, *Cremation of Amputated Parts of the Body, and of Fetuses*, March 7, 1967

7

Sacred Rites of the Church and Practices Concerning the Sick

Holy Communion

92. What are the guidelines for the reception of Holy Communion if one is ill?

[Can. 918] It is highly recommended that the faithful receive Holy Communion during the Eucharistic Celebration itself. It is to be administered outside the Mass, however, to those who request it for a just cause, with the liturgical rites being observed.

[Can. 919] §1 A person who is to receive the Most Holy Eucharist is to abstain for at least one hour before Holy Communion from any food and drink, except for only water and medicine. . . .

§3 The elderly, the infirm, and those who care for them can receive the Most Holy Eucharist even if they have eaten something within the preceding hour.

—Code of Canon Law, cc. 918, 919 §§1, 3

[Can. 921] §1 The Christian faithful who are in danger of death from any cause are to be nourished by Holy Communion in the form of Viaticum.

§2 Even if they have been nourished by Holy Communion on the same day, however, those in danger of death are strongly urged to receive Communion again.

113

§3 While the danger of death lasts, it is recommended that Holy Communion be administered often, but on separate days.

[Can. 922] Holy Viaticum for the sick is not to be delayed too long; those who have the care of souls are to be zealous and vigilant that the sick are nourished by Viaticum while fully conscious.

—*Code of Canon Law*, cc. 921–922

The Sunday Obligation

93. What about obligations for attending Mass when one is ill?

On Sundays and other holy days of obligation, the faithful are obliged to participate in the Mass. Moreover, they are to abstain from those works and affairs which hinder the worship to be rendered to God, the joy proper to the Lord's Day, or the suitable relaxation of mind and body.

—*Code of Canon Law*, c. 1247

If participation in the Eucharistic Celebration becomes impossible because of the absence of a sacred minister or for another grave cause, it is strongly recommended that the faithful take part in a Liturgy of the Word if such a liturgy is celebrated in a parish church or other sacred place according to the prescripts of the diocesan bishop or that they devote themselves to prayer for a suitable time alone, as a family, or, as the occasion permits, in groups of families.

—*Code of Canon Law*, c. 1248 §2

Since the Eucharist is the very heart of Sunday, it is clear why, from the earliest centuries, the pastors of the Church have not ceased to remind the faithful of *the need to take part in the liturgical assembly*. "Leave everything on the Lord's Day," urges the third-century text known as the *Didascalia*, "and run diligently to your assembly, because it is your praise of God. Otherwise, what excuse will they make to God, those who do not come together on the Lord's Day to hear the word of life and feed on the divine nourishment which lasts forever?" The faithful have generally accepted this call of the pastors with conviction of soul and, although there have been times and situations when this duty has not been perfectly met, one should never forget the genuine heroism of priests and faithful who have fulfilled this obligation even when faced with danger and the denial of religious freedom, as can be documented from the first centuries of Christianity up to our own time.

In his first *Apology* addressed to the Emperor Antoninus and the Senate, Saint Justin proudly described the Christian practice of the Sunday assembly, which gathered in one place Christians from both the city and the countryside. When, during the persecution of Diocletian, their assemblies were banned with the greatest severity, many were courageous enough to defy the imperial decree and accepted death rather than miss the Sunday Eucharist. This was the case of the martyrs of Abitina, in Proconsular Africa, who replied to their accusers: "Without fear of any kind we have celebrated the Lord's Supper, because it cannot be missed; that is our law"; "We cannot live without the Lord's Supper." As she confessed her faith, one of the martyrs said: "Yes, I went to the assembly and I celebrated the Lord's Supper with my brothers and sisters, because I am a Christian."

Even if in the earliest times it was not judged necessary to be prescriptive, the Church has not ceased to confirm this obligation of conscience, which rises from the inner need felt so strongly by the Christians of the first centuries. It was only later, faced with the half-heartedness or negligence of some, that the Church had to make explicit the duty to attend Sunday Mass: more often than not, this was done in the form of exhortation, but at times the Church had to resort to specific canonical precepts. This was the case in a number of local councils from the fourth century onwards (as at the Council of Elvira of 300, which speaks not of an obligation but of penalties after three absences) and most especially from the sixth century onwards (as at the Council of Agde in 506). These decrees of local councils led to a universal practice, the obligatory character of which was taken as something quite normal.

The Code of Canon Law of 1917 for the first time gathered this tradition into a universal law. The present code reiterates this, saying that "on Sundays and other holy days of obligation the faithful are bound to attend Mass." This legislation has normally been understood as entailing a grave obligation: this is the teaching of the *Catechism of the Catholic Church*, and it is easy to understand why if we keep in mind how vital Sunday is for the Christian life.

Today, as in the heroic times of the beginning, many who wish to live in accord with the demands of their faith are being faced with difficult situations in various parts of the world. They live in surroundings which are sometimes decidedly hostile and at other times—more frequently in fact—indifferent and unresponsive to the Gospel message. If believers

115

are not to be overwhelmed, they must be able to count on the support of the Christian community. This is why they must be convinced that it is crucially important for the life of faith that they should come together with others on Sundays to celebrate the Passover of the Lord in the sacrament of the New Covenant. It is the special responsibility of the bishops, therefore, "to ensure that Sunday is appreciated by all the faithful, kept holy and celebrated as truly 'the Lord's Day,' on which the Church comes together to renew the remembrance of the Easter mystery in hearing the word of God, in offering the sacrifice of the Lord, in keeping the day holy by means of prayer, works of charity, and abstention from work" [Sacred Congregation for Bishops, *Directory for the Pastoral Ministry of Bishops*, 86a].

Because the faithful are obliged to attend Mass unless there is a grave impediment, Pastors have the corresponding duty to offer to everyone the real possibility of fulfilling the precept. The provisions of Church law move in this direction, as for example in the faculty granted to priests, with the prior authorization of the diocesan bishop, to celebrate more than one Mass on Sundays and holy days, the institution of evening Masses and the provision which allows the obligation to be fulfilled from Saturday evening onwards, starting at the time of First Vespers of Sunday. From a liturgical point of view, in fact, holy days begin with First Vespers. Consequently, the liturgy of what is sometimes called the "Vigil Mass" is in effect the "festive" Mass of Sunday, at which the celebrant is required to preach the homily and recite the Prayer of the Faithful.

Moreover, pastors should remind the faithful that when they are away from home on Sundays they are to take care to attend Mass wherever they may be, enriching the local community with their personal witness. At the same time, these communities should show a warm sense of welcome to visiting brothers and sisters, especially in places which attract many tourists and pilgrims, for whom it will often be necessary to provide special religious assistance.

—John Paul II, *Dies Domini*, 46–49

Sunday, on which by apostolic tradition the Paschal Mystery is celebrated, must be observed in the universal Church as the primordial holy day of obligation. The following days must also be observed: the Nativity of our Lord Jesus Christ, the Epiphany, the Ascension, the Body and Blood of Christ, Holy Mary the Mother of God, her Immaculate

Conception, her Assumption, Saint Joseph, Saint Peter and Saint Paul the Apostles, and All Saints.

—*Code of Canon Law*, c. 1246 §1

Care of the Dying

94. What does the Church offer pastorally for the care of the dying?

A privileged moment of prayer with the terminally ill person is the celebration of the *sacraments*: being signs of God's saving presence, "Penance, the Anointing of the Sick, and the Eucharist as viaticum constitute at the end of Christian life 'the sacraments that prepare for our heavenly homeland' or the sacraments that complete the earthly pilgrimage."

In particular, in the sacrament of *Reconciliation* or *Penance*, the dying person, at peace with God, is at peace with himself and with his neighbor.

"In addition to the Anointing of the Sick, the Church offers those who are about to leave this life the Eucharist as viaticum." Received at this moment of passage, the Eucharist, as viaticum, is the sacrament of "passing over" from death to life, from this world to the Father, and it gives the dying person the strength to confront the final, decisive stage of his journey in life. It follows that it is important for the Christian to request it, and it is also a duty of the Church to administer it. The minister of viaticum is the priest. If no priest is available, it may be conferred by the deacon or, in his absence, by an extraordinary minister of the Eucharist.

—Pontifical Council for Pastoral Assistance to Health Care Workers,
New Charter for Health Care Workers, 163
(quoting *Catechism of the Catholic Church*, 1525, 1524)

All baptized Christians who can receive communion are obliged to receive viaticum, if in danger of death from any cause. Pastors must ensure that the administration of this sacrament is not delayed, but that it is made available to the faithful while they are still in possession of their faculties.

—Congregation for Divine Worship,
The Rite of Anointing and Pastoral Care of the Sick, 27

95. What are the guidelines for the sacrament of the Anointing of the Sick?

[Can. 998] The anointing of the sick, by which the Church commends the faithful who are dangerously ill to the suffering and glorified Lord in order that he relieve and save them, is conferred by anointing them with oil and pronouncing the words prescribed in the liturgical books.

[Can. 999] In addition to a bishop, the following can bless the oil to be used in the anointing of the sick: those equivalent to a diocesan bishop by law; any presbyter in a case of necessity, but only in the actual celebration of the sacrament.

[Can. 1000] *§1* The anointings with the words, order, and manner prescribed in the liturgical books are to be performed carefully. In a case of necessity, however, a single anointing on the forehead or even on some other part of the body is sufficient, while the entire formula is said.

§2 The minister is to perform the anointings with his own hand, unless a grave reason warrants the use of an instrument.

[Can. 1001] Pastors of souls and those close to the sick are to take care that the sick are consoled by this sacrament at the appropriate time.

[Can. 1002] The communal celebration of the anointing of the sick for many of the sick at once, who have been suitably prepared and are properly disposed, can be performed according to the prescripts of the diocesan bishop.

[Can. 1003] §1 Every priest and a priest alone validly administers the anointing of the sick.

§2 All priests to whom the care of souls has been entrusted have the duty and right of administering the anointing of the sick for the faithful entrusted to their pastoral office. For a reasonable cause, any other priest can administer this sacrament with at least the presumed consent of the priest mentioned above.

§3 Any priest is permitted to carry blessed oil with him so that he is able to administer the sacrament of the anointing of the sick in a case of necessity.

[Can. 1004] §1 The anointing of the sick can be administered to a member of the faithful who, having reached the use of reason, begins to be in danger due to sickness or old age.

§2 This sacrament can be repeated if the sick person, having recovered, again becomes gravely ill or if the condition becomes more grave during the same illness.

[Can. 1005] This sacrament is to be administered in a case of doubt whether the sick person has attained the use of reason, is dangerously ill, or is dead.

[Can. 1006] This sacrament is to be conferred on the sick who at least implicitly requested it when they were in control of their faculties.

[Can. 1007] The anointing of the sick is not to be conferred upon those who persevere obstinately in manifest grave sin.

—Code of Canon Law, cc. 998–1007

96. In cases of imminent death of an unbaptized person, who can administer the Sacrament of Baptism?

When an ordinary minister is absent or impeded, a catechist or another person designated for this function by the local ordinary, or in a case of necessity any person with the right intention, confers baptism licitly.

—Code of Canon Law, c. 861 §2

An adult in danger of death can be baptized if, having some knowledge of the principal truths of the faith, the person has manifested in any way at all the intention to receive baptism and promises to observe the commandments of the Christian religion.

—Code of Canon Law, c. 865 §2

§1 Parents are obliged to take care that infants are baptized in the first few weeks; as soon as possible after the birth or even before it, they are to go to the pastor to request the sacrament for their child and to be prepared properly for it.

§2 An infant in danger of death is to be baptized without delay.

—Code of Canon Law, c. 867

An infant of Catholic parents or even of non-Catholic parents is baptized licitly in danger of death even against the will of the parents.

—Code of Canon Law, c. 868 §2

97. Where can one find formal common prayers and devotional practices for the sick and for healing?

See Congregation for Divine Worship, *Pastoral Care of the Sick: Rites of Anointing and Viaticum.*

98. What is World Day of the Sick?

Welcoming the request you have made, as president of the Pontifical Council for the Pastoral Care of Health Workers, and also as an interpreter of the expectation of many episcopal conferences and national and international Catholic bodies, I would like to inform you that I have decided to establish the "World Day of the Sick," to be celebrated on February 11 of each year, the liturgical memorial of the Blessed Virgin Mary of Lourdes....

The annual celebration of the "World Day of the Sick" therefore has the manifest purpose of raising awareness among the People of God and, consequently, the multiple Catholic health institutions and civil society itself, of the need to ensure the best assistance to the sick; to help those who are ill to value suffering, on the human level and above all on the supernatural level; to involve in a particular way dioceses, Christian communities, religious families in health care; to foster the increasingly valuable commitment of volunteering; to recall the importance of the spiritual and moral formation of health workers and, finally, to better understand the importance of religious assistance to the sick by diocesan and regular priests, as well as by those who live and work alongside those who suffer.

—John Paul II, Letter to Cardinal Fiorenzo Angelini, President of the Pontifical Council for Pastoral Care for Health Workers, for the Establishment of the World Day of the Sick, May 13, 1992, 1–2

The World Day of the Sick—in its preparation, realization and objectives—is not meant to be reduced to a mere external display centering on certain initiatives, however praiseworthy they may be, but is intended to reach consciences to make them aware of the valuable contribution which human and Christian service to those suffering makes to better understanding among people and, consequently, to building real peace.

Indeed, peace presupposes, as its preliminary condition, that special attention be reserved for the suffering and the sick by public authorities, national and international organizations, and every person of good will. This is valid, first of all, for developing countries—in Latin America, Africa and Asia—which are marked by serious deficiencies in health care. With the celebration of the World Day of the Sick, the Church is promoting a renewed commitment to those populations, seeking to wipe out the injustice existing today by devoting greater human, spiritual, and material resources to their needs.

In this regard, I wish to address a special appeal to civil authorities, to people of science, and to all those who work in direct contact with the sick. May their service never become bureaucratic and aloof! Particularly, may it be quite clear to all that the administration of public money imposes the serious duty of avoiding its waste and improper use so that available resources, administered wisely and equitably, will serve to ensure prevention of disease and care during illness for all who need them.

The hopes which are so alive today for a humanization of medicine and health care require a more decisive response. To make health care more humane and adequate it is, however, essential to draw on a transcendent vision of man which stresses the value and sacredness of life in the sick person as the image and child of God. Illness and pain affect every human being: love for the suffering is the sign and measure of the degree of civilization and progress of a people.

—John Paul II, Message for the First Annual
World Day of the Sick, October 21, 1992, 4

8

Medical Research

99. What values does the Church recognize as constituting medical research practice?

Scientific knowledge has its own value in the domain of medical science. . . . Knowledge as such and the full understanding of any truth raise no moral objection. By virtue of this principle, research and the acquisition of truth for arriving at new, wider, and deeper knowledge and understanding of the same truth are in themselves in accordance with the moral order.

But this does not mean that all methods, or any single method, arrived at by scientific and technical research offers every moral guarantee. . . . Sometimes it happens that a method cannot be used without injuring the rights of others or without violating some moral rule of absolute value. In such a case, although one rightly envisages and pursues the increase of knowledge, morally the method is not admissible. Why not? Because science is not the highest value. . . . Science itself, therefore, as well as its research and acquisitions, must be inserted in the order of values. Here there are well-defined limits which even medical science cannot transgress without violating higher moral rules. The confidential relations between doctor and patient, the personal right of the patient to the life of his body and soul in its psychic and moral integrity are just some of the many values superior to scientific interest.

—Pius XII, "*The Moral Limits of Medical Research and Treatment*," September 14, 1952, 7–8

No person, moreover, may be used thoughtlessly as an object for the purpose of therapeutic experimentation; therapeutic experimentation must take place in accordance with protocols that respect fundamental ethical norms. Every treatment or process of experimentation must be with a view to possible improvement of the person's physical condition and *not merely seeking scientific advances.*

—Benedict XVI, Address to Members of the International Congress of Catholic Pharmacists, October 29, 2007 (emphasis added)

Catholics should be among the first to support scientists in their fidelity to goals that enhance and promote life. Catholics, and especially Catholic scientists, must bear a special witness, standing firm to defend the basic dignity of the human person.

—USCCB, *Health and Health Care,* IV.B.2

100. What are the ethical norms that determine what research is permissible?

The ethical norms of research require that it be directed toward promoting human well-being. All research contrary to the true good of the person is immoral; investing efforts and resources in it is contrary to the human purpose of science and scientific progress.

—Pontifical Council for Pastoral Assistance to Healthcare Workers, *New Charter for Health Care Workers,* 100

I would like to repeat here what I already wrote some time ago: Here there is a problem that we cannot get around; no one can dispose of human life. An insurmountable limit to our possibilities of doing and of experimenting must be established. The human being is not a disposable object, but every single individual represents God's presence in the world.

—Benedict XVI, Address to the Participants in the Symposium on the Theme: "Stem Cells: What Future for Therapy?" September 16, 2006

In the *experimentation* phase, or the testing of a research study's hypotheses on human beings, the good of the person—protected by ethical norms—demands respect for preconditions connected essentially with consent and risk.

—Pontifical Council for Pastoral Assistance to Healthcare Workers, *New Charter for Health Care Workers,* 100

EDITOR'S NOTE: The various aspects of risk are further explained immediately below, and the issue of consent is addressed further below. ✤

101. Is there a degree of risk that is by itself a reason against doing the research, even if the patient may consent to it?

First is the *risk factor*. In itself all experimentation involves some risks. However, "there is a degree of danger that morality cannot allow." There is a threshold beyond which the risk becomes humanly unacceptable. This threshold is defined by the inviolable good of the person, which forbids all concerned "to endanger his life, his equilibrium, his health, or to aggravate his illness."

—Pontifical Council for Pastoral Assistance to Healthcare Workers,
New Charter for Health Care Workers, 101 (quoting Pius XII, "The Moral Limits of
Medical Research and Treatment," September 14, 1952; and John Paul II, Address
to an International Conference on Pharmacy, October 24, 1986, 4)

Research or experimentation on the human being cannot legitimate acts that are in themselves contrary to the dignity of persons and to the moral law. The subjects' potential consent does not justify such acts. Experimentation on human beings is not morally legitimate if it exposes the subject's life or physical and psychological integrity to disproportionate or avoidable risks.

—*Catechism of the Catholic Church*, 2295

As for the patient, he is not absolute master of himself, of his body or of his soul. He cannot, therefore, freely dispose of himself as he pleases. Even the reason for which he acts is of itself neither sufficient nor determining. The patient is bound to the immanent teleology laid down by nature. He has the right of use, limited by natural finality, of the faculties and powers of his human nature....

The patient, then, has no right to involve his physical or psychic integrity in medical experiments or research when they entail serious destruction, mutilation, wounds, or perils.

—Pius XII, "*The Moral Limits of Medical Research and Treatment*,"
September 14, 1952, 13–14

Where does the doctor find a moral limit in research into and use of new methods and procedures in the "interests of the patient?" The limit is the same as that for the patient. It is that which is fixed by the judgment of sound reason, which is set by the demands of the natural moral law, which is deduced from the natural teleology inscribed in beings and from the scale of values expressed by the nature of things. The limit is the same for the doctor as for the patient because, as We have already said, the doctor as a private individual disposes only of the rights given him by the patient and because the patient can give only what he himself possesses.

—Pius XII, "*The Moral Limits of Medical Research and Treatment*,"
September 14, 1952, 18

102. What degree of risk is permissible if a competent patient consents to it?

Without doubt, before giving moral authorization to the use of new methods, one cannot ask that any danger or any risk be excluded.... In doubtful cases, when means already known have failed, it may happen that a new method still insufficiently tried offers, together with very dangerous elements, appreciable chances of success. If the patient gives his consent, the use of the procedure in question is licit. But this way of acting cannot be upheld as a line of conduct in normal cases.

—Pius XII, "*The Moral Limits of Medical Research and Treatment*,"
September 14, 1952, 38

If there are no other sufficient remedies, it is permitted, with the patient's consent, to have recourse to the means provided by the most advanced medical techniques, even if these means are still at the experimental stage and are not without a certain risk. By accepting them, the patient can even show generosity in the service of humanity.

—Congregation for the Doctrine of the Faith,
Declaration on Euthanasia, IV

Experimentation cannot be initiated and continued unless all precautions have been taken to avoid foreseeable risks and to reduce the consequences of adverse outcomes....

Once these guarantees are met, in the *clinical phase*, human experimentation must abide by the *principle of proportionate risk*, that is, of a due proportion between foreseeable harms and benefits.

—Pontifical Council for Pastoral Assistance to Healthcare Workers,
New Charter for Health Care Workers, 102

103. Why does the Church require informed consent to participate in research experimentation?

Experimentation on human beings does not conform to the dignity of the person if it takes place without the informed consent of the subject or those who legitimately speak for him.

—*Catechism of the Catholic Church*, 2295

The consent of the subject is needed. He "must be informed of the experimentation, of its purpose and any risks it involves, so that he may give or refuse his consent in full awareness and freedom. The doctor, in fact, has only that power and those rights over the patient which the patient himself confers to him."

—Pontifical Council for Pastoral Assistance to Healthcare Workers,
New Charter for Health Care Workers, 103 (quoting John Paul II, Address to
Participants in Two Congresses on Medicine and Surgery, 5)

The properly documented *provision of adequate information and verification of understanding*, for the purposes of obtaining free and cognizant consent from the persons involved, are always a necessary and indispensable element for *ethical experimentation*, both when the objectives are strictly for scientific knowledge and when these are connected with additional objectives involving therapeutic potential.

—Pontifical Council for Pastoral Assistance to Healthcare Workers,
New Charter for Health Care Workers, 101

104. If consent is necessary, is research on children or adults not capable of making decisions (hereafter the non-consenting) not permissible?

Minors or adults who are legally not capable of understanding and making decisions can also be involved in clinical experimentation, provided that, subject to the criteria of scientific validity, their involvement is justified by a proportionality between the reasonably foreseeable risks and benefits for the minor or incapacitated subjects.

—Pontifical Council for Pastoral Assistance to Healthcare Workers,
New Charter for Health Care Workers, 101

In clinical experimentation, *presumed consent* can be taken into consideration only in the case of an experimental procedure to be carried out in an urgent or emergency situation on patients who are not capable of understanding and deciding and are suffering from a pathology for which the experimental procedure is the sole possibility for treatment and the experimentation has been approved previously by an ethics committee. Later the patient, if he regains competence (or his legal representative if the patient's incapacity persists), must be informed about the experimentation and either confirm his participation or not (deferred consent).

—Pontifical Council for Pastoral Assistance to Healthcare Workers,
New Charter for Health Care Workers, 104

105. Is research permissible if there is not an expected benefit from the proposed research on the non-consenting?

Experimentation that is not expected to provide direct benefits for the minor or incapacitated subjects, but only for other persons in similar conditions (in terms of age, type of illness, and other characteristics), can be ethically justified when it is not possible to obtain the same results through experiments on adult, competent subjects and the risks and burdens are minimal. In both cases, informed consent must be requested of the parents or the legal representative in accordance with the laws of each particular country.

—Pontifical Council for Pastoral Assistance to Healthcare Workers,
New Charter for Health Care Workers, 101

106. Are there added moral conditions for research on sick patients?

In *experimentation on a sick person for therapeutic purposes*, due proportion must be attained by comparing the conditions of the sick person with the possible clinical benefits of the experimental drugs or methods. The evaluation of the risks must be done in advance by the researcher and by the ethics committee, and this is a fundamental aspect of the ethical justification for any clinical experimentation. For this evaluation, the already-stated principle applies: "If there are no other sufficient remedies, it is permitted, with the patient's consent, to have recourse to the means provided by the most advanced medical techniques, even if these means are still at the experimental stage and are not without a certain risk. By accepting them, the patient can even show generosity in the service of humanity."

—Pontifical Council for Pastoral Assistance to Healthcare Workers,
New Charter for Health Care Workers, 104 (quoting Congregation for the
Doctrine of the Faith, *Declaration on Euthanasia*, IV)

107. Are there specific conditions for research on vulnerable persons, including research in developing countries?

In clinical experimentation, moreover, special attention must be given to the involvement of *persons* who may be *vulnerable* because of dependence (students, prisoners, military service personnel), social insecurity or poverty (the homeless, the unemployed, immigrants), or lack of education, which could make it difficult to obtain valid informed consent.

In emerging and developing countries, experimentation should have first and foremost clinical and scientific objectives that directly and specifically concern the local populations involved. *The scientific and ethical criteria used to evaluate and conduct the experiments in emerging and developing countries must be the same as those used for experimentation conducted in developed countries* [emphasis added].

Experiments in emerging and developing countries must be conducted with respect to local traditions and cultures and should be approved in advance by either a national ethics committee of the sponsoring country or by the local ethics committee.

—Pontifical Council for Pastoral Assistance to Healthcare Workers,
New Charter for Health Care Workers, 107

108. Are there specific conditions for permitting research on healthy persons who are not in need of any therapy?

Clinical experimentation can be carried out also *on a healthy person* who voluntarily offers himself "to contribute by his initiative to the progress of medicine and, in that way, to the good of the community." This is legitimized by human and Christian solidarity, which justifies the gesture and gives it meaning and value: "To give something of oneself, within the limits laid down by the moral norm, may constitute a highly meritorious witness of charity and an occasion of spiritual growth so significant as to be able to compensate for the risk of a slight physical disability." In any case, it is always necessary to interrupt the experimentation if intermediate evaluations indicate an excessive risk or a clear lack of benefit.

—Pontifical Council for Pastoral assistance to Healthcare Workers, *New Charter for Health Care Workers*, 105 (quoting John Paul II, Address to Participants in Two Congresses on Medicine and Surgery, 5)

109. Is it permissible to use animals for research purposes?

Experimentation cannot be initiated and continued unless all precautions have been taken to avoid foreseeable risks and to reduce the consequences of adverse outcomes.

To obtain these assurances, a phase of basic *preclinical research* is necessary, which must provide the fullest documentation and the surest guarantees about pharmacological toxicology and operating techniques. To this end, if useful and necessary, experimentation with new drugs or new techniques cannot exclude the *use of animals* before going on to human subjects. "It is certain that animals are at the service of man and can hence be the object of experimentation. Nevertheless, they must be treated as creatures of God which are destined to serve man's good, but not to be abused by him." It follows that all experimentation "should be carried out with consideration for the animal, without causing it useless suffering."

—Pontifical Council for Pastoral Assistance to Health Care Workers, *New Charter for Health Care Workers*, 102 (quoting John Paul II, Address to Members of the Pontifical Academy of Sciences, 4; and Address to an International Conference on Pharmacy, October 24, 1986, 4)

110. Is medical research on infertility permissible?

Research for diagnosing the condition and appropriate treatment is the correct scientific approach to the question of infertility, and also the one that best respects the integral humanity of those involved. Indeed, the union of the man and the woman in the community of love and life, which is marriage, constitutes the only worthy "place" to call into existence a new human being, who is always a gift.

—Benedict XVI, Address to Participants in the General Assembly of the Pontifical Academy for Life, February 25, 2012.

111. Is it morally permissible to perform therapeutic surgery on pre-born human beings?

As with all medical interventions on patients, *one must uphold as licit procedures carried out on the human embryo which respect the life and integrity of the embryo and do not involve disproportionate risks for it but are directed towards its healing, the improvement of its condition of health, or its individual survival.* Whatever the type of medical, surgical, or other therapy, the free and informed consent of the parents is required, according to the deontological rules followed in the case of children.

—Congregation for the Doctrine of the Faith, *Donum vitae,* I.3

A strictly therapeutic intervention whose explicit objective is the healing of various maladies such as those stemming from chromosomal defects will, in principle, be considered desirable, provided it is directed to the true promotion of the personal well-being of the individual without doing harm to his integrity or worsening his conditions of life. Such an intervention would indeed fall within the logic of the Christian moral tradition.

—John Paul II, Address at the Conclusion of the Thirty-fifth General Assembly of the World Medical Association, October 29, 1983

112. Is medical research on pre-born human beings permissible?

Medical research must refrain from operations on live embryos, unless there is a moral certainty of not causing harm to the life or integrity of the unborn child and the mother, and on condition that the parents have given their free and informed consent to the procedure. It follows that all research, even when limited to the simple observation of the embryo, would become illicit were it to involve risk to the embryo's physical integrity or life by reason of the methods used or the effects induced.... *If the embryos are living, whether viable or not, they must be respected just like any other human person; experimentation on embryos which is not directly therapeutic is illicit.*

—Congregation for the Doctrine of the Faith, *Donum vitae,* I.4

113. Is it morally permissible to do non-therapeutic research on pre-born human beings?

EDITOR'S NOTE: In one sense, all research is non-therapeutic since the goal is to acquire knowledge, knowledge about *whether or not* a drug, device, or procedure is beneficial. What the Church means by non-therapeutic research is research that does not take into account or recognize the good of the individual research subject. So, even high-risk research on consenting adults can be problematic on the Church's view. This is clarified further in answer to question 114 below. ✣

Nontherapeutic experiments on a living embryo or fetus are not permitted, even with the consent of the parents. Therapeutic experiments are permitted for a proportionate reason with the free and informed consent of the parents or, if the father cannot be contacted, at least of the mother. Medical research that will not harm the life or physical integrity of an unborn child is permitted with parental consent.

—USCCB, *Ethical and Religious Directives for Catholic Health Care Services*, 51

Proposals to *use these embryos for research* or *for the treatment of disease* are obviously unacceptable because they treat the embryos as mere "biological material" and result in their destruction. The proposal to thaw such embryos without reactivating them and use them for research, as if they were normal cadavers, is also unacceptable.

—Congregation for the Doctrine of the Faith, *Dignitas personae*, 19

EDITOR'S NOTE: "These embryos" refers to embryos that were conceived in vitro but not transferred to the mother's uterus and thereafter frozen. ✣

I condemn, in the most explicit and formal way, experimental manipulations of the human embryo, since the human being, from conception to death, cannot be exploited for any purpose whatsoever.

—John Paul II, Address to a Meeting of the Pontifical Academy of Sciences, October 23, 1982, 4

Respect for the dignity of the human being excludes all experimental manipulation or exploitation of the human embryo.

—Pontifical Council for the Family, *Charter of the Rights of the Family*, 4b

Any form of experimentation on the fetus that may damage its integrity or worsen its condition is unacceptable, except in the case of a final effort to save it from death.

—John Paul II, Address to the Participants in the Convention
of the Pro-Life Movement, December 3, 1982

114. In general, is therapeutic research on pre-born human beings permissible?

Medical research must refrain from operations on live embryos, unless there is a moral certainty of not causing harm to the life or integrity of the unborn child and the mother, and on condition that the parents have given their free and informed consent to the procedure. It follows that all research, even when limited to the simple observation of the embryo, would become illicit were it to involve risk to the embryo's physical integrity or life by reason of the methods used or the effects induced.... *If the embryos are living, whether viable or not, they must be respected just like any other human person; experimentation on embryos which is not directly therapeutic is illicit.* No objective, even though noble in itself, such as a foreseeable advantage to science, to other human beings or to society, can in any way justify experimentation on living human embryos or fetuses, whether viable or not, either inside or outside the mother's womb....

... In the case of experimentation that is clearly therapeutic, namely, when it is a matter of experimental forms of therapy used for the benefit of the embryo itself in a final attempt to save its life, and in the absence of other reliable forms of therapy, recourse to drugs or procedures not yet fully tested can be licit.

—Congregation for the Doctrine of the Faith, *Donum vitae*, I.4

115. Is it immoral for a medical researcher to endorse the use of oral contraceptive drugs or other contraceptive products for subjects in research if, for example, the drug being tested might harm a developing human being?

EDITOR'S NOTE: Here is a case in which, according to the Introduction, a work outside of the ordinary (and extraordinary) Magisterium is used. In this case, it is used for all three reasons, namely, no clear teaching already exists, but what is said here is still reflective of the mind of the Church, and the guidance is informative. For context, anytime there is medical research, there must be informed consent (and child-bearing women should be able to provide consent). One way in which that consent is procured is through an informed consent document that explains the research and what is going to be done to the person. For example, if one is testing a drug that is dangerous to developing human beings, one should not get pregnant during the study. Therefore, can a researcher *recommend*, or *endorse*, the use of artificial contraceptives to prevent harm to a developing child? ✛

A. Subjects should not be required to use contraception. However, subjects can be required to take appropriate precautions to avoid pregnancy or fathering a child. The level of certainty with which pregnancy is to be avoided may be specified in the protocol.

B. The subjects must be free to choose how they will avoid pregnancy or father a child, although as noted above the level of certainty may be specified.

C. It is permissible to convey information to subjects on the effectiveness of various methods of pregnancy prevention, and verify their understanding, as long as it is clear that use of contraceptives is not required. Conveying information but not requiring contraception is not immoral cooperation because the writer or health professional is providing factual information that is in the public domain, which is morally different than advocating or encouraging the use of contraception.

D. Abstinence should always be included as an acceptable method for avoiding pregnancy or fathering a child.

E. Certain methods of preventing pregnancy may be prohibited. For example, birth control pills may be prohibited in studies where drug interactions with oral contraceptives could occur and pose a safety risk, or otherwise alter the outcome of the study.

F. Abortion is never permissible as a method of birth control.

—The Catholic Medical Association and the National Catholic Bioethics Center, "A Catholic Guide to Ethical Clinical Research," Principle 3, Case 3.1, 207–8 (reformatted for readability)

9

Conflicts of Interest

116. What does the Church teach about conflicts of interest; what are they and what are their sources?

In advanced societies, research, and specifically biomedical research, is one of the most far-reaching and dynamic fields of innovation and progress, drawing investment both from public bodies and from private groups, often of a multinational character.

While it is certainly proper for a firm in the field of biomedical or pharmaceutical research to seek an appropriate return on investment, it sometimes happens that overriding financial interests prompt decisions and products which are contrary to truly human values and to the demands of justice, demands which cannot be separated from the very aim of research. As a result, a conflict can arise between economic interests on the one hand and, on the other, medicine and health-care. Research in this field must be pursued for the good of all, including those without means.

—John Paul II, Letter to Msgr. Jozef Kowalczyk participating in the international conference on "Conflicts of Interest and Its Significance in Science and Medicine," March 25, 2002

The Church respects and supports scientific research when it has a genuinely humanist orientation, avoiding any form of instrumentalization or destruction of the human being and keeping itself free from the slavery of political and economic interests.

—John Paul II, Address to the Members of the Pontifical Academy for Life, February 24, 2003, 4

117. What are the possible effects of not monitoring conflicts of interest in health care?

There is a risk that science-based businesses and healthcare structures can be set up not in order to provide the best possible care for people in accordance with their human dignity, but in order to maximize profits and increase business, with a predictable lowering in the quality of service for those unable to pay.

—John Paul II, Letter to Msgr. Jozef Kowalczyk Participating in the International Conference on "Conflicts of Interest and Its Significance in Science and Medicine," March 25, 2002

118. What are some specific ways in which these conflicts manifest themselves in medical research?

The selection of research programs, where those programs which hold out the promise of a quick profit are often preferred to other research which involves higher costs and a greater investment of time because it respects the demands of ethics and justice. Driven by the pursuit of profit and catering to what could be called "the medicine of desires," the pharmaceutical industry has favored research which has already placed on the world market products contrary to the moral good, including products which are not respectful of procreation and even suppress human life already conceived. . . .

Another example of such conflict of interest is the way in which priorities are set for pharmaceutical research. In developed countries, for instance, huge sums are spent on producing medicines that serve hedonistic purposes, or in marketing different brands of already available and equally effective medicines; while in poorer areas of the world, drugs are not available for the treatment of devastating and deadly diseases. In these countries access to even the most basic medicines is almost impossible because the profit motive is absent. Likewise, in the case of certain uncommon diseases the industry offers no financial support for research and the production of medicines, because there is no prospect of profits: these are the so-called orphan drugs.

—John Paul II, Letter to Msgr. Jozef Kowalczyk Participating in the International Conference on "Conflicts of Interest and Its Significance in Science and Medicine," March 25, 2002

119. What is the Church's guidance on how to minimize conflicts of interest in medical research and clinical practice?

For science to retain its true independence and for researchers to retain their freedom, ethical values must be brought to the fore. . . .

For scientific research in the biomedical field to be restored to its full dignity, researchers themselves must be fully engaged. It is primarily up to them to guard jealously and, if necessary, to reclaim the essential meaning of that mastery and dominion over the visible world which the Creator entrusted to man as a task and duty. As I wrote in my first encyclical letter *Redemptor hominis*, this meaning "consists in the priority of ethics over technology, in the primacy of the person over things, and in the superiority of spirit over matter." Consequently, I added, "all phases of present-day progress must be followed attentively. Each stage of that progress must, so to speak, be x-rayed from this point of view"

—John Paul II, Letter to Msgr. Jozef Kowalczyk Participating in the International Conference on "Conflicts of Interest and Its Significance in Science and Medicine," March 25, 2002

10

The Role of Physicians, and the Patient–Physician Relationship

120. Considering the autonomy of a patient, shouldn't a physician have a moral obligation to provide whatever treatment or medical procedure that a patient may wish?

Health care is carried out in everyday practice in an interpersonal relationship characterized by the trust of a person who is experiencing suffering and sickness, who has recourse to the knowledge and conscience of a healthcare worker who encounters him in order to support and care for him, thus adopting a sincere attitude of "com-passion," in the etymological sense of the word [i.e., to suffer with].

Such a relationship with the sick person, with full respect for his autonomy, requires availability, attention, understanding, empathy, and dialogue, together with expertise, competence, and professional ethics. That is to say, it must be the expression of a profoundly human commitment, made and carried out not just as a technical activity but as an act of dedication and love of neighbor.

Service to life is performed only in *fidelity to the moral law*, which expresses its value and duties. Indeed, for the healthcare worker there are moral responsibilities too, the guidelines for which spring from bioethical reflection. In this field, with vigilant, zealous attention, the magisterium of the Church makes pronouncements in reference to the questions raised by biomedical progress and by the changeable cultural *ethos*.

For the healthcare worker, this magisterium is a source of principles and norms of behavior, which enlightens his conscience and orients it—especially in the complexity of today's biotechnological possibilities—toward decisions that always respect the human person and his dignity. Through fidelity to the moral norm, the healthcare worker lives out his fidelity to man, whose value the norm safeguards, and to God, whose wisdom the norm expresses.

Advances in medicine and the constant appearance of new moral questions, therefore, require on the part of the healthcare worker a serious *preparation and ongoing formation* in order to maintain the necessary professional competence. To this end it is desirable that all healthcare workers be suitably trained and that those responsible for their professional formation endeavor to establish professorial chairs and courses in bioethics. Furthermore, in the principal hospital centers, the establishment of ethics committees for medical practice and clinical ethics services should be promoted. In them medical competence and evaluation meet and are integrated with the competence of other professionals who are attending the sick person, to safeguard the dignity of the patient and medical responsibility itself.

—Pontifical Council for Pastoral Assistance to Health Care Workers, *New Charter for Health Care Workers*, 4–5

When the law permits abortion, healthcare workers "must refuse politely but firmly." A human being can never obey an intrinsically immoral law, as is the case with a law that admitted, as a matter of principle, that abortion is licit. The force of the inviolability of human life and of God's law, which defends it, precedes any positive human law. When human law contradicts it, conscience affirms its primary right and the primacy of God's law: "We must obey God rather than men" (Acts 5:29).

—Pontifical Council for Pastoral Assistance to Health Care Workers, *New Charter for Health Care Workers*, 59 (quoting John Paul II, Address to the Participants in a Meeting for Obstetricians, January 26, 1980)

121. What does the spirit have to do with the body? Shouldn't a doctor focus on the body only and leave the spiritual to somebody else?

The activity of healthcare workers, in their complementary roles and responsibilities, has the value of service to the human person, since to protect, recover, and improve physical, psychological, and spiritual health means to serve life in its totality.

—Pontifical Council for Pastoral Assistance to Health Care Workers,
New Charter for Health Care Workers, 2

122. Are there Church guidelines about praying with patients?

The *spiritual crisis* evoked as death draws near prompts the Church to become for the dying person and his family the bearer of the light of hope, which only faith can shine on the mystery of death. Death is an event that introduces one into God's life, about which only revelation can pronounce a word of truth. The proclamation of the Gospel, which is "full of grace and truth" (Jn 1:14), accompanies the Christian from the beginning to the end of life—which conquers death—and opens human dying to the greatest hope.

It is therefore necessary to give an *evangelical meaning to death*: proclaiming the Gospel to the dying person. This is a pastoral duty of the ecclesial community in all its members, according to each one's responsibilities. A particular task belongs to the healthcare chaplain, who is called in a singular way to provide pastoral care for the dying within the broader scope of his care for the sick.

For him this task involves not only the personal role at the bedside of the dying persons entrusted to his care, but also the promotion of this pastoral work in terms of the organization of religious services, training and sensitizing healthcare workers and volunteers, as well as involving relatives and friends. The expressive forms of the proclamation of the Gospel to the dying person are charity, prayer, and the sacraments.

—Pontifical Council for Pastoral Assistance to Health Care Workers,
New Charter for Health Care Workers, 159–60

123. Do physicians participate in the process of canonization of saints?

In the case of miraculous healings, the physicians who treated the patient are to be called as witnesses.

If they refuse to appear before the bishop or his delegate, the aforementioned is to see to it that they write a report, sworn if possible, about the disease and its progress, which is to be inserted into the acts, or at least their opinion is to be heard by a third party, who is then to be examined.

In their testimony, which is to be sworn to under oath, the witnesses must indicate the source of their knowledge of the things they assert; otherwise, their testimony is to be considered of no value.

If any witness prefers to give to the bishop or his delegate a previously prepared written statement, either together with his deposition or in addition to it, such a written statement is to be accepted, provided the witness himself shall have proved by an oath that he himself wrote it and that its contents are true. It is also to be made part of the acts of the cause. . . .

In the case of a cure from some disease, the bishop or his delegate is to seek help from a physician, who is to propose questions to the witnesses in order to clarify matters according to necessity and circumstances.

If the person healed is still alive, he is to be examined by experts so that the duration of the healing can be ascertained.

—Congregation for the Causes of Saints, "Norms to Be Observed in the Inquiries Made by Bishops in the Causes of Saints," February 7, 1983, 22–24, 34

It should not be forgotten that in the examination of events claimed to be miraculous the competence of scholars and theologians converges, although the last word is given to theology, the only discipline that can give a miracle an interpretation of faith.

This is why the process of saints' causes moves from the scientific evaluation of the medical council or technical experts to a theological examination by the consultors and later by the cardinals and bishops. Moreover, it should be clearly borne in mind that the uninterrupted practice of the Church establishes the need for a *physical* miracle, since a moral miracle does not suffice.

—Benedict XVI, Letter to the Participants of the Plenary Session of the Congregation for the Causes of Saints, April 24, 2006

The miracle, required for the Beatification of the Venerable Servants of God and for the Canonization of the Blessed, was always examined with the utmost rigor. Already in medieval times recourse was made to medical experts for whom, on September 17, 1743, a specific register was created by Benedict XIV. More recently, Pius XII established a Commission of Doctors at the Congregation of the Sacred Rites on October 20, 1948, to which he added, on December 15, 1948, a special Medical Council.

John XXIII, on July 10, 1959, unified these two bodies into a Medical Council, approving the Regulations . In the light of new requirements and on the basis of the Apostolic Constitution *Sacra Rituum Congregatio* of May 8, 1969, a further revision of the norms of the Regulations was carried out, which was approved by Paul VI on April 23, 1976.

The promulgation of the Apostolic Constitution *Divinus perfectionis Magister* by John Paul II, on January 25, 1983, and the experience of this Congregation in recent years highlighted the need to update again the Regulations of the Medical Council.

For this purpose, the following norms of the Regulations of the Medical Council of the Congregation for the Causes of Saints have been drawn up.

—Congregation for the Causes of Saints, "Regulations of the Medical Council of the Congregation for the Causes of Saints," September 23, 2016, introduction

11

Love Manifested
in Social Justice

124. Is health care considered a human right by the Church?

The first right of the human person, the right to life, entails a right to the means for the proper development of life, such as adequate health care.

—USCCB, *Ethical and Religious Directives
for Catholic Health Care Services*, Part One, introduction

First We must speak of man's rights. Man has the right to live. He has the right to bodily integrity and to the means necessary for the proper development of life, particularly food, clothing, shelter, medical care, rest, and, finally, the necessary social services.

—John XXIII, *Pacem in terris*, 11

The fundamental right to the preservation of health pertains to the *value of justice*, whereby there are no distinctions between peoples and ethnic groups, taking into account their objective living situations and stages of development, in pursuing the *common good*, which is at the same time the good of all and of each individual.

—Pontifical Council for Pastoral Assistance to Health Care Workers,
New Charter for Health Care Workers, 141

The political community has a duty to honor the family, to assist it, and to ensure especially: . . . *in keeping with the country's institutions*, the right to medical care, assistance for the aged, and family benefits.

—*Catechism of the Catholic Church*, 2211 (emphasis added)

Today, health care is recognized as a universal human right and as an essential dimension of integral human development. However, at [a] global level, it still remains a right guaranteed to the few and unavailable to many.

—Francis, Address to Participants in the Symposium Promoted by the Somos Community Care Organization, September 20, 2019

Healthcare workers and their professional associations in particular are called to this task [i.e., addressing global health inequities], since they are committed to raising awareness among institutions, welfare agencies, and the healthcare industry as a whole, for the sake of ensuring that every individual actually benefits from the *right to health care.*

—Francis, Message to the Participants in the Thirty-second International Conference on "Addressing Global Health Inequalities," November 18, 2017 (emphasis added)

The right to life is the *right to live with human dignity,* in other words, to be guaranteed this fundamental, original, and inalienable good, which is the root and prerequisite for every other right of the human person, and to have this good safeguarded.

"The human being is entitled to such rights, *in every phase of development,* from conception until natural death; and *in every condition,* whether healthy or sick, whole or handicapped, rich or poor."

—Pontifical Council for Pastoral Assistance to Health Care Workers, *New Charter for Health Care Workers,* 63 (quoting John Paul II, *Christifideles laici,* 38)

The fundamental and primary right of every human being to life, which more particularly entails the right to the protection of health, takes priority over the *labor union rights of healthcare workers.*

—Pontifical Council for Pastoral Assistance to Health Care Workers, *New Charter for Health Care Workers,* 66

In effect the acknowledgment of the personal dignity of every human being demands *the respect, the defense, and the promotion of the rights of the human person.* It is a question of inherent, universal, and inviolable rights. No one, no individual, no group, no authority, no State, can change—let alone eliminate—them because such rights find their source in God himself.

The inviolability of the person which is a reflection of the absolute inviolability of God, finds its primary and fundamental expression in the *inviolability of human life*. Above all, the common outcry, which is justly made on behalf of human rights—for example, the right to health, to home, to work, to family, to culture—is false and illusory if *the right to life*, the most basic and fundamental right and the condition for all other personal rights, is not defended with maximum determination.

—John Paul II, *Christifideles laici*, 38

The sick person deserves treatments that are possible and from which he may derive some benefit. Indeed, every human being has a primary right to what is necessary for the maintenance of his own health and therefore to *adequate health care*. Consequently, those who care for the sick have the duty to carry out their work with the utmost diligence and to provide any treatments considered necessary or useful. This includes not only those that aim at a possible recovery, but also palliative treatments that relieve pain and ease an incurable condition. In this regard it is necessary to use special caution in resorting to treatments that lack documentation of scientific validity.

—Pontifical Council for Pastoral Assistance to Health Care Workers,
New Charter for Health Care Workers, 85

125. Who is responsible for ensuring that this right is realized and respected?

Although institutions that provide these services [healthcare] are very important, no institution can by itself replace the human heart or human compassion when it is a matter of encountering the sufferings of another.

—Pontifical Council for Pastoral Assistance to Health Care Workers,
New Charter for Health Care Workers, 3

The government, working for the common good, has an essential role to play in assuring that the right of all people to adequate health care is protected.

—USCCB, *Health and Health Care*, V

126. What basic values should guide the formation of a national health policy?

The Dignity of the Human Person

Catholic healthcare ministry is rooted in a commitment to promote and defend human dignity; this is the foundation of its concern to respect the sacredness of every human life from the moment of conception until death.

—USCCB, *Ethical and Religious Directives*
for Catholic Health Care Services, Part One, introduction

Every person has a basic right to adequate health care. This right flows from the sanctity of human life and the dignity that belongs to all human persons, who are made in the image of God.

—USCCB, *Health and Health Care*, V.1

Preferential Option for the Poor

The biblical mandate to care for the poor requires us to express this in concrete action at all levels of Catholic health care.... In Catholic institutions, particular attention should be given to the healthcare needs of the poor, the uninsured, and the underinsured.

—USCCB, *Ethical and Religious Directives*
for Catholic Health Care Services, Part One, introduction

[Human dignity and the sanctity of human life imply] that access to that health care which is necessary and suitable for the proper development and maintenance of life must be provided for all people, regardless of economic, social, or legal status. Special attention should be given to meeting the basic health needs of the poor. Special attention should be given to meeting the basic health needs of the poor. With increasingly limited resources in the economy, it is the basic rights of the poor that are frequently threatened first.

—USCCB, *Health and Health Care*, V, 1

Genuine healthcare reform must especially focus on the basic health needs of the poor.

—USCCB, *A Framework for Comprehensive Health Care Reform*

Commitment to the Common Good

Catholic healthcare ministry seeks to contribute to the common good. The common good is realized when economic, political, and social conditions ensure protection for the fundamental rights of all individuals and enable all to fulfill their common purpose and reach their common goals.

—USCCB, *Ethical and Religious Directives for Catholic Health Care Services*, Part One, introduction

Stewardship

Catholic healthcare ministry exercises responsible stewardship of available healthcare resources. A just healthcare system will be concerned both with promoting equity of care—to assure that the right of each person to basic health care is respected—and with promoting the good health of all in the community.

—USCCB, *Ethical and Religious Directives for Catholic Health Care Services*, Part One, introduction

The benefits provided in a national healthcare policy should be sufficient to maintain and promote good health as well as to treat disease and disability. Emphasis should be placed on the promotion of health, and prevention of disease, and the protection against environmental and other hazards to physical and mental health.

—USCCB, *Health and Health Care*, V, 3

Public policy should ensure that uniform standards are part of the healthcare delivery system.

—USCCB, *Health and Health Care*, V, 5

Incentives should be developed at every level for administering health care efficiently, effectively, and economically.

—USCCB, *Health and Health Care*, V, 6

Pluralism and the Right of Conscience

Catholic health care does not offend the rights of individual conscience by refusing to provide or permit medical procedures that are judged morally wrong by the teaching authority of the Church.

—USCCB, *Ethical and Religious Directives for Catholic Health Care Services*, Part One, introduction

149

Pluralism is an essential characteristic of the healthcare delivery system of the United States. Any comprehensive health system that is developed, therefore, should use the cooperative resources of both the public and private sectors, the voluntary, religious, and non-profit sectors.

—USCCB, *Health and Health Care*, V, 2

Consumers should be allowed a reasonable choice of providers.

—USCCB, *Health and Health Care*, V, 4

127. Is it permissible to support healthcare policies that promise to provide quality and universally accessible health care if they include funding for abortion or euthanasia or other contra-life actions?

We strongly believe it would be morally wrong and counterproductive to compel individuals, institutions, or states to pay for or participate in procedures that fundamentally violate basic moral principles and the consciences of millions of Americans. The common good is not advanced when advocates of so-called choice compel taxpayers to fund what we and many others are convinced is the destruction of human life.

—USCCB, *A Framework for Comprehensive Health Care Reform*

128. Do pharmaceutical companies have an obligation to distribute scarce resources such as vaccines?

Finally, there is also a moral imperative for the pharmaceutical industry, governments, and international organizations *to ensure that vaccines, which are effective and safe from a medical point of view, as well as ethically acceptable, are also accessible to the poorest countries in a manner that is not costly for them.* The lack of access to vaccines, otherwise, would become another sign of discrimination and injustice that condemns poor countries to continue living in health, economic, and social poverty.

—Congregation for the Doctrine of the Faith,
Note on the Morality of Using Some Anti-COVID-19 Vaccines, 6

The issue of production is also linked to that of *vaccine patents.* The financing of research has followed different paths, in the form of both the investment of resources from States (issued directly to research, or though prior purchase of a certain number of doses), and donations from private entities. It is therefore a matter of specifying how the vaccine can effectively become a "common good," as already expressed by several political leaders (e.g., the president of the European Commission). In fact, since it is not an existing natural resource (such as air or oceans), nor a discovery (such as the genome or other biological structures), but an invention produced by human ingenuity, it is possible to subject it to economic consideration, which allows the recovery of the research costs and risks companies have taken on. Nonetheless, given its function, it is appropriate to consider the vaccine as a good to which everyone should have access, without discrimination, according to the principle of the universal destination of goods highlighted by Pope Francis. "We [cannot] allow the virus of radical individualism to get the better of us and make us indifferent to the suffering of other brothers and sisters . . . letting the law of the marketplace and patents take precedence over the law of love and the health of humanity."

—Pontifical Academy for Life, "Vaccine for All: 20 Points for a Fairer and Healthier World," 7 (quoting Pope Francis, *Urbi et orbi*, December 25, 2020)

Those who live in poverty are poor in everything, even medicines, and therefore their health is more vulnerable. Sometimes they run the risk of not being able to obtain treatment because of lack of money, or because some people in the world do not have access to certain medicines. There is also a "pharmaceutical marginality," and this must be said. This creates a further gap between nations and between peoples. On an ethical level, if there is the possibility of curing a disease with a drug, it should be available to everyone, otherwise it creates injustice. Too many people, too many children are still dying in the world because they are denied access to a drug that is available in other regions, or a vaccine. We know the danger of the globalization of indifference. Instead, I propose to globalize treatment, that is, the possibility of access to those drugs that could save so many lives for all populations. And to do this takes a joint effort, a convergence that involves everyone.

—Francis, Address to the Members of the "Banco farmaceutico" Foundation, September 19, 2020

Today, in this time of darkness and uncertainty regarding the pandemic, various lights of hope appear, such as the discovery of vaccines. But for these lights to illuminate and bring hope to all, they need to be available to all. We cannot allow the various forms of nationalism closed in on themselves to prevent us from living as the truly human family that we are. Nor can we allow the virus of radical individualism to get the better of us and make us indifferent to the suffering of other brothers and sisters. I cannot place myself ahead of others, letting the law of the marketplace and patents take precedence over the law of love and the health of humanity. I ask everyone—government leaders, businesses, international organizations—to foster cooperation and not competition, and to seek a solution for everyone: vaccines for all, especially for the most vulnerable and needy of all regions of the planet. Before all others: the most vulnerable and needy!

—Francis, Urbi et orbi, December 25, 2020

129. Do pharmaceutical companies or device manufacturers have an obligation to distribute healthcare resources to the poor?

The development of economic activity and growth in production are meant to provide for the needs of human beings. Economic life is not meant solely to multiply goods produced and increase profit or power; it is ordered first of all to the service of persons, of the whole man, and of the entire human community.

—Catechism of the Catholic Church, 2426

Those responsible for business enterprises are responsible to society for the economic and ecological effects of their operations. They have an obligation to consider the good of persons and not only the increase of profits.

—Catechism of the Catholic Church, 2432

Healthcare strategies aimed at pursuing justice and the common good must be economically and ethically sustainable. Indeed, while they must safeguard the sustainability both of research and of healthcare systems, at the same time they ought to make available essential drugs in adequate quantities, in usable forms of guaranteed quality, along with correct information, and at costs that are affordable by individuals and communities.

—Pontifical Council for Pastoral Assistance to Health Care Workers,
New Charter for Health Care Workers, 92

It would also be advisable that the different pharmaceutical firms, laboratories at hospital centers and surgeries, as well as our contemporaries all together, be concerned with showing solidarity in the therapeutic context, to make access to treatment and urgently needed medicines available at all levels of society and in all countries, particularly to the poorest people."

—Benedict XVI, Address to Members of the International Congress of Catholic Pharmacists, October 29, 2007

There is an increasingly urgent need to fill *the very serious and unacceptable gap* that separates the developing world from the developed in terms of the capacity to develop biomedical research for the benefit of healthcare assistance and to assist peoples afflicted by chronic poverty and dire epidemics....

It is essential to realize that to leave these peoples without the resources of science and culture means to condemn them to poverty, financial exploitation, and the lack of healthcare structures, and also to commit an injustice and fuel a long-term threat for the globalized world. To value endogenous human resources means to guarantee the balance of health care and, in short, to contribute to the peace of the whole world. Thus the relevant moral dimension of biomedical scientific research necessarily opens to the dimension of justice and international solidarity.

—John Paul II, Address to the Members of the Pontifical Academy for Life, February 24, 2003, 6

130. Does the State (government) have an obligation to facilitate distribution of healthcare resources?

It is the task of the State to provide for the defense and preservation of common goods such as the natural and human environments, which cannot be safeguarded simply by market forces. Just as in the time of primitive capitalism the State had the duty of defending the basic rights of workers, so now, with the new capitalism, the State and all of society have the duty of *defending those collective goods* which, among others, constitute the essential framework for the legitimate pursuit of personal goals on the part of each individual.

—John Paul II, *Centesimus annus*, 40

Private agencies and institutions alone are unable to develop a comprehensive national health policy, or to ensure that all Americans have adequate health insurance, or to command the vast resources necessary to implement an effective national health policy. These functions are in large part the responsibility of government.

—USCCB, *Health and Health Care*, V

131. Do pharmaceutical companies have an obligation to do research and development on treatments for rare but debilitating diseases?

EDITOR'S NOTE: Rare diseases are defined as diseases that occur in the population at a particular time in very low frequency. For example, the European Union defines the frequency of rare diseases at 1/10,000 persons. ✢

Although it cannot be denied that the scientific knowledge and research of *pharmaceutical companies* have their own laws by which they must abide—for example, the protection of intellectual property and a fair profit to support innovation—ways must be found to combine these adequately with the right of access to basic or necessary treatments, or both, especially in underdeveloped countries, and above all in the cases of so-called *rare* and *neglected diseases*, which are accompanied by the notion of *orphan drugs*.

—Pontifical Council for Assistance to Healthcare Workers,
New Charter for Health Care Workers, 92

Study, research, and technology applied to life and health must, in fact, be factors of growth for all humanity, in solidarity with and respect for the dignity of every human person, especially the weak and defenseless.

—John Paul II, Address to an International
Healthcare Conference, November 8, 1997, 4

The Church does not forget her smallest children and if, on the one hand she applauds the initiatives of the richer nations to improve the conditions of their development, on the other, she is strongly aware of the need to invite them to pay greater attention to these brothers and sisters of ours, so that thanks to our unanimous solidarity they are able to look at life with trust and hope.

—Benedict XVI, Address to the Participants in the 23rd International Congress
Organized by the Pontifical Council for Health Pastoral Care, November 15, 2008

132. In the setting of scarce resources, is there an established order of preference as to who may receive the resource?

When there is a question of allocating scarce resources, the vulnerable and the poor have a compelling claim to first consideration. Special attention must be given to ensuring that those who have suffered from inaccessible and inadequate health care . . . are first brought back into an effective system of quality care.

—USCCB, *A Framework for Comprehensive Health Care Reform*

In the public debate, there are different positions on the criteria of *administration* and *access* to the vaccine. Despite the difference, however, we find certain lines of convergence that we intend to support. There is agreement on the priority to be given to professional categories engaged in services of common interest, in particular health personnel. This also includes activities that require contact with the public (such as school and public security), vulnerable groups (such as the elderly, or people with particular pathologies). Of course, such a criterion does not resolve all situations. A grey area remains, for example, when defining the priorities of vaccine implementation within the very same risk group. A more attentive stratification of populations could help resolve these dilemmas (e.g., vaccine in areas with higher density maximizes its benefits). In addition, other relevant aspects besides health (such as the different practicability of restrictive measures) for a fair distribution must be taken into account.

This *order of administration*, at an international level, implies that "the priority must be given to vaccinating . . . some people in all countries, rather than all people in some countries." That some countries receive the vaccine late due to prior large-scale purchase by richer states must be avoided. It is a question of agreeing on the specific percentages according to which to concretely proceed. Vaccine *distribution* requires a number of *tools* that must be specified and implemented to achieve the agreed objectives in terms of universal accessibility criteria.

—Pontifical Academy for Life, "Vaccine for All: 20 Points for a Fairer and Healthier World," 11–12 (quoting WHO Director Tedros Ghebreyesus, August 18, 2020)

133. What is the moral responsibility for pharmaceutical companies and other healthcare sector businesses regarding economic market forces?

The sole purpose of commercial exploitation is not ethically acceptable in the field of medicine and health care. Investments in the medical field should find their deepest meaning in human solidarity. For this to happen, we ought to identify appropriate systems that favor transparency and cooperation, rather than antagonism and competition.

—Pontifical Academy for Life,
"Vaccine for All: 20 Points for a Fairer and Healthier World," 8

In fact, the purpose of a business firm is not simply to make a profit, but is to be found in its very existence as a *community of persons* who in various ways are endeavoring to satisfy their basic needs, and who form a particular group at the service of the whole of society. Profit is a regulator of the life of a business, but it is not the only one; *other human and moral factors* must also be considered which, in the long term, are at least equally important for the life of a business.

—John Paul II, *Centesimus annus*, 35

134. What is the moral obligation to vote, particularly when healthcare issues are the subject of laws and policies affecting a society?

Those who are involved in healthcare policy and financial administrators have a responsibility not only to their specific fields, but also toward society and the sick.

It is up to them, in particular, to defend and promote the common good, performing the duty of justice, according to the principles of solidarity and subsidiarity, in developing national and worldwide policies aimed at the authentic development of peoples, especially in the allocation of financial resources in the healthcare field.

In this light, those responsible for healthcare policies can bring about fruitful collaboration by acknowledging the distinctive character of Catholic healthcare facilities, thereby contributing to the building of "the 'civilization of love and life,' without which the life of individuals and of society itself loses its most genuinely human quality."

—Pontifical Council for Pastoral Assistance to Health
Care Workers, *New Charter for Health Care Workers*, 7
(quoting John Paul II, *Evangelium vitae*, 27)

Suggestions for Further Reading

Magisterial Documents and Episcopal Teaching Documents:

These documents are available on the Vatican or United States Conference of Catholic Bishops websites, unless otherwise noted.

Benedict XVI. Letter to the Participants of the Plenary Session of the Congregation for the Causes of Saints. April 24, 2006.

———. Address to the Participants in the Symposium on the Theme "Stem Cells: What Future for Therapy?" September 16, 2006.

———. Address to Members of the International Congress of Catholic Pharmacists. October 29, 2007.

———. Address to the Participants in the Twenty-Third International Congress Organized by the Pontifical Council for Health Pastoral Care. November 15, 2008.

———. Encyclical Letter. *Caritas in veritate*. June 29, 2009.

———. Address to Participants in the General Assembly of the Pontifical Academy for Life. February 25, 2012.

Catechism of the Catholic Church. 2nd ed. Translated by United States Conference of Catholic Bishops. Vatican City: Libreria Editrice Vaticana, 1997.

Code of Canon Law. 1983.

Congregation for the Doctrine of Faith. *Declaration on Procured Abortion*. November 18, 1974.

———. *Persona humana* (On Certain Questions Concerning Sexual Ethics). December 29, 1975.

———. *Quaecumque sterilizatio*, Reply of the Sacred Congregation for the Doctrine of the Faith on Sterilization and Catholic Hospitals. March 13, 1975.

———. *Declaration on Euthanasia*. May 5, 1980.

———. *Donum vitae*. February 22, 1987.

———. *Responses to Certain Questions of the United States Conference of Catholic Bishops Concerning Artificial Nutrition and Hydration*. August 1, 2007.

———. *Dignitas personae*, On Certain Bioethical Questions. June 20, 2008.

———. "Principles for Collaboration with Non-Catholic Entities." *National Catholic Bioethics Quarterly* 14, no. 2 (2014): 337–40.

———. *Response to a Question on the Liceity of a Hysterectomy in Certain Cases*. January 3, 2019.

———. *Samaritanus bonus* (On the Care of Persons in the Critical and Terminal Phases of Life). September 22, 2020.

———. Note on the Morality of Using Some Anti-COVID-19 Vaccines. December 21, 2020.

John Paul II. Apostolic Exhortation. *Familiaris consortio*. November 22, 1981.

———. Apostolic Letter. *Salvifici doloris*. February 11, 1984.

———. Apostolic Letter *"Motu proprio." Dolentium hominum*. February 11, 1985.

———. Apostolic Letter. *Mulieris dignitatem*. August 15, 1988.

———. Encyclical Letter. *Centesimus annus*. May 1, 1991.

———. Encyclical Letter. *Veritatis splendor*. August 6, 1993.

———. Encyclical Letter. *Evangelium vitae*. March 25, 1995.

———. Apostolic Letter. *Dies Domini*. May 31, 1998.

———. Address to the Eighteenth International Congress of the Transplantation Society. August 29, 2000.

———. Address to the Participants in the International Congress on Life-Sustaining Treatments and Vegetative State: Scientific Advances and Ethical Dilemmas. March 20, 2004.

John XXIII. Encyclical Letter. *Pacem in terris*. April 11, 1963.

Leo XIII. Encyclical Letter. *Libertas praestantissimum* (On the Nature of Human Liberty). June 20 1888.

Paul VI. Encyclical Letter. *Humanae vitae*, On the Regulation of Birth. July 25, 1968.

Pius X. Encyclical Letter. *Singulari quadam*. September 24, 1912.

Pius XI. Encyclical Letter. *Casti connubii*. December 31, 1930.

Pius XII. Encyclical Letter. *Humani generis*. August 12, 1950.

———. "The Moral Limits of Medical Research and Treatment." Address to the Participants in the First International Congress on Histopathology of the Nervous System. September 14, 1952. https://www.papalencyclicals.net/pius12/p12psych.htm.

———. "Morality and Eugenics." Address to the Participants in the Seventh Congress of the International Society of Hematology. September 12, 1958. *The Pope Speaks* 6, no. 4 (1960): 392–400.

Pontifical Council for Pastoral Assistance to Health Care Workers. *New Charter for Health Care Workers.* Translated by National Catholic Bioethics Center. Philadelphia: National Catholic Bioethics Center, 2017.

Pontifical Council for the Family. *Charter of the Rights of the Family.* October 22, 1983.

United States Conference of Catholic Bishops (USCCB). *Ethical and Religious Directives for Catholic Health Care Services.* 6th ed. Washington, DC: USCCB, 2018.

Vatican Council II. *Dignitatis humanae.* Declaration on Religious Liberty. December 7, 1965.

———. *Gaudium et spes.* Pastoral Constitution on the Church in the Modern World. December 7, 1965.

Select Works by Authors and Research Institutes

What follows is a list of select articles and studies. For a comprehensive list of works on Catholic clinical bioethics, consult the bibliographies of Furton, *Catholic Health Care Ethics: A Manual for Practitioners,* 3rd ed.; and Ashley, O'Rourke, and DeBlois, *Health Care Ethics: A Catholic Theological Analysis,* 5th ed. Both are cited in full below.

Anscombe Bioethics Centre (formerly the Linacre Centre for Healthcare Ethics). "Human Dignity, Autonomy and Mentally Incapacitated Persons: A Response to Who Decides?" 1998. https://www.bioethics.org.uk/research/reports-submissions/human-dignity-autonomy-and-mentally-incapacitated-persons/.

Aquinas. Thomas. *Summa theologiae.* Translated by the Fathers of the English Dominican Province. New York: Benziger Brothers, 1948.

Ashley, B.M., K.D. O'Rourke, and J. DeBlois. *Health Care Ethics: A Catholic Theological Analysis.* 5th ed. Washington, DC: Georgetown University Press, 2006.

Ballentine, Jennifer, Cordt Kassner, and Ira Byock. "Physician-Assisted Death Does Not Improve End-of-Life Care." *Journal of Palliative Medicine* 19 (2016): 479–80.

Cataldo, P.J., and J.M. Haas. "Institutional Cooperation: The ERDs." *Health Progress* 83, no. 6 (2002): 49–57.

Charlotte Lozier Institute. "Assisted Suicide Is Not Compassion." April 28, 2015. https://lozierinstitute.org/assisted-suicide-is-not-compassion/.

Condic, M.L. "When Does Human Life Begin: The Scientific Evidence and Terminology Revisited." *University of St. Thomas Journal of Law & Public Policy* 8 (2013): 44–81.

———. "A Biological Definition of the Human Embryo." In *Persons, Moral Worth, and Embryos*, edited by Stephen Napier, 211–35. Dordrecht: Springer Publishers, 2011.

———. "When Does Human Life Begin? A Scientific Perspective." *Westchester Institute White Paper* 1, no. 1 (2008): 1–18.

Coope, C.M. "Death with Dignity." *The Hastings Center Report* 27, no. 5 (1997): 37–39.

Furton, E.J., ed. *Catholic Health Care Ethics: A Manual for Practitioners*, 3rd ed. Philadelphia: National Catholic Bioethics Center, 2022.

Gormally, Luke, ed. *Euthanasia, Clinical Practice and the Law*. London: The Linacre Centre for Health Care Ethics, 1994.

Keown, John. *Euthanasia, Ethics and Public Policy: An Argument against Legalization*. Cambridge: Cambridge University Press, 2018.

Lee, Tara Sander, Maria B. Feeney, Kathleen M. Schmainda, James L. Sherley, and David A. Prentice. "Human Fetal Tissue from Elective Abortions in Research and Medicine: Science, Ethics, and the Law." *Issues in Law & Medicine* 35 (2020): 3–60.

Napier, Stephen. *Uncertain Bioethics: Moral Risk and Human Dignity*. New York: Routledge, 2019.

National Catholic Bioethics Center and the Catholic Medical Association. "A Catholic Guide to Ethical Clinical Research." *The Linacre Quarterly* 75, no. 3 (2008): 181–224.

O'Brien, Dan, John Paul Slosar, and Anthony R. Tersigni. "Utilitarian Pessimism, Human Dignity, and the Vegetative State: A Practical Analysis of the Papal Allocution." *The National Catholic Bioethics Quarterly* 4, no. 3 (2004): 497–512.

Pike, Gregory. "The Provision of Nutrition and Hydration to Vulnerable Patients: An Analysis of the Clinical and Ethical Issues." 2019. Bios Centre. https://bioscentre.org/wp-content/uploads/2019/10/Nutrition_and_hydration_for_vulnerable_patients_GPike_web.pdf.

———. "Euthanasia and Assisted Suicide—When Choice Is an Illusion and Informed Consent Fails." 2020. Bios Centre. https://bioscentre.org/articles/euthanasia-and-assisted-suicide-when-choice-is-an-illusion-and-informed-consent-fails/.

Pontifical Academy for Life. "Vaccine for All: 20 Points for a Fairer and Healthier World." December 29, 2020. https://www.vatican.va/roman_curia/pontifical_academies/acdlife/documents/rc_pont-acd_life_doc_20201229_covid19-vaccinopertuttti_en.html.

———. "Moral Reflections on Vaccines Prepared from Cells Derived from Aborted Human Foetuses." 2005. *Linacre Quarterly* 86, nos. 2–3 (2019): 182–87.

———. *Prospects for Xenotransplantation: Scientific Aspects and Ethical Considerations.* 2001. https://www.vatican.va/roman_curia/pontifical_academies/acdlife/documents/rc_pa_acdlife_doc_20010926_xenotrapianti_en.html.

Prentice, David. "Update: COVID-19 Vaccine Candidates and Abortion-Derived Cell Lines." June 2, 2021. Charlotte Lozier Institute. https://lozierinstitute.org/update-covid-19-vaccine-candidates-and-abortion-derived-cell-lines/.

Sánchez Sorondo, Marcelo. *Signs of Death.* Vatican City: Pontifical Academy of the Sciences, 2007.

Tarne, Eugene. "Human Embryonic Stem Cell Research 25 Years on." October 30, 2023. Charlotte Lozier Institute. https://lozierinstitute.org/human-embryonic-stem-cell-research-25-years-on/.

Watt, Helen. *Life and Death in Healthcare Ethics: A Short Introduction.* London: Routledge, 2000.

White, R.J., H. Angstwurm, and C. De Paula, eds. *The Determination of Brain Death and Its Relationship to Human Death.* Vatican City: Pontifical Academy of the Sciences, 1992.

Relevant and Informative Websites

Anscombe Bioethics Centre (formerly the Linacre Centre for Healthcare Ethics). https://www.bioethics.org.uk/

The Bios Centre. https://bioscentre.org/.

The Bioethics Defense Fund. https://bdfund.org/.

The Center for Bioethics and Culture Network. https://cbc-network.org/.

The Center for Bioethics and Human Dignity. https://www.cbhd.org/.

The Charlotte Lozier Institute. https://lozierinstitute.org/.

The National Catholic Bioethics Center (NCBC). https://www.ncbcenter.org/.

Also from The Catholic University of America Press

Catholic Witness in Health Care: Practicing Medicine in Truth and Love
Edited by John M. Travaline and Louise A. Mitchell

Biomedicine and Beatitude: An Introduction to Catholic Bioethics, second edition
by Nicanor Pier Giorgio Austriaco, OP

Pellegrino's Clinical Bioethics: A Compendium
by Edmund D. Pellegrino
Edited by G. Kevin Donovan, David G. Miller and Claudia Ruiz Sotomayor

*A Catechism for Business: Tough Ethical Questions & Insights
from Catholic Teaching*, third edition
Edited by Andrew V. Abela and Joseph E. Capizzi

*A Catechism for Family Life: Insights from Catholic Teaching
on Love, Marriage, Sex, and Parenting*
Edited by Sarah Bartel and John S. Grabowski

Handbook of Catholic Social Teaching: A Guide for Christians in the World Today
Edited by Martin Schlag

Available at cuapress.org
from the National Catholic Bioethics Center

Handbook on Critical Life Issues, fourth edition
by Arland K. Nichols

Catholic Health Care Ethics: A Manual for Practitioners, third edition
by Edward J. Furton

New Charter for Health Care Workers, English edition
by Pontifical Council for Pastoral Assistance to Health Care Workers

Courage Through Chronic Disease: Discovery, Hope, Transformation
by Carolyn Humphreys

The Art of Dying
by Br. Columba Thomas, OP, MD

Transgender Issues in Catholic Health Care
by Edward J. Furton

Life is a Blessing: A Biography of Jérôme Lejeune—Geneticist, Doctor, Father
by Clara Lejeune-Gaymard